Brewer
Arthritis Sourcebook
31369

C —
616.7
B

MAR 2 0 1999

DATE DUE

JUN 13, 2008	
DISCARDED	
	PRINTED IN U.S.A.

THE ARTHRITIS SOURCEBOOK

THE ARTHRITIS SOURCEBOOK

Everything You Need to Know About:

- *The major types of arthritis and their treatments*
- *Building your treatment team*
- *Medications and alternative therapies*
- *Exercise and nutrition*
- *Sleep problems and sex*
- *Assistive devices*
- *Special issues such as employment, surgery, and pregnancy*

Earl J. Brewer, Jr., M.D.

and

Kathy Cochran Angel

Lowell House
Los Angeles
Contemporary Books
Chicago

Library of Congress Cataloging-in-Publication Data

Brewer, Earl J., 1928–
     The arthritis sourcebook : everything you need to know / Earl J. Brewer, Jr.,
     and Kathy Cochran Angel.
          p.   cm.
     Includes bibliographical references and index.
     ISBN 1-56565-036-0
     1. Arthritis—Popular works. I. Angel, Kathy Cochran. II. Title.

RC933.B725 1993
616.7'22—dc20   92-39063
                                                                 CIP

Requests for such permissions should be addressed to:
Lowell House
2029 Century Park East, Suite 3290
Los Angeles, CA 90067
Publisher: Jack Artenstein
Executive Vice-President: Nick Clemente
Vice-President/Editor-in-Chief: Janice Gallagher
Director of Publishing Services: Mary D. Aarons
Text Design: Mary Ballachino

Manufactured in the United States of America
10 9 8 7 6 5 4 3 2 1

Contents

Part 3: *Taking Care of Yourself*

Part 4: *Paying Attention to Your Special Issues*

Dedication

To Ria, still the best of the best.
With such apparent ease she makes everything possible.

E. J. B.

To my family and to the many families
whose lives have been touched by arthritis,
and especially to Gary, my best friend and partner.

K. C. A.

Acknowledgments

To the many patients with arthritis who graciously gave of their time to tell what they would like to see in an arthritis sourcebook. In particular, Mr. John Carrabba and Mrs. Virginia Ray were extremely helpful.

To Rick Benzel, our editor. His flexibility and excellent suggestions added greatly to the book. I (EJB) learned a great deal from him.

To David Taylor, exercise trainer, for listening and offering many good suggestions to help people with arthritis.

To Gay Koenning, nutritionist and team coordinator, for her help with nutrition.

To Joy Cordery, occupational therapist, for lending a sympathetic ear as well as advice about what is and is not important to people with arthritis.

To medical colleagues Michael Weinblatt, Thomas Thornhill, James Cassidy, Ted Pincus, Leigh Callahan, Rollie Moskawitz, James Kemper, and John Sergent, for advice and knowledge about people with arthritis and for feedback on the manuscript.

To Alice Brandfonbrener for sharing her experiences concerning artists who have arthritis.

And last, to Pat Jones for advice and help in getting things done for many years.

Preface

Living Well in the Face of Arthritis

A Note from Kathy

This is a book about one of the most pervasive diseases this country is facing today. An estimated 37,000,000 people are affected by one of the more than 100 types of arthritis, and one family in three is impacted by this disease. Symptoms range from those much advertised "minor aches and pains of arthritis" to serious, life-threatening problems.

I presume you are reading this book because you have arthritis or someone you love has arthritis. If so, you know firsthand how this disease pervades every aspect of your life. It is not just a physical struggle but a mental and emotional one as well. Chronic pain is a most debilitating fact in daily living. In order to live life to the fullest, you need to gain control over this nemesis. One way to do that is by closely observing those people who have been successful in their attempts and by avoiding the mistakes of those who have not.

Arthritis has been a thread woven throughout my life. One of my earliest memories is of my grandmother, Ruth, a role model in the very best sense of the word. She taught me so many beautiful things, things only a grandmother could have the time to teach. She taught me to crochet, to do needlepoint, to sew—things that required tremendous manual dexterity. It was only as an adult that I realized that during the time we spent together she was ignoring the pain of rheumatoid arthritis. In her time, medical thinking was to put people with arthritis to bed. But as a widow raising five children alone, she did not have time for that. She simply continued her daily tasks to the best of her abilities, took buffered aspirin for the pain, and rested when she could. This was fortunate for her, because as we now know the best possible approach to arthritis is to keep moving at all costs. Today's physicians encourage people with arthritis to remain as active as possible in order to maintain muscle strength. My grandmother was a courageous woman and living life to the fullest was much more important to her than the pain in her joints. It was more important to share her talents with her grandchildren than to give in to a disease that would not leave her in peace. After she finally had to enter a nursing home, in a wheelchair, she continued giving generously of herself by teaching her fellow residents to play the piano, sharing the beauty she saw in life.

Her daughter, my aunt, was diagnosed at the age of 27 with the same rheumatoid arthritis. It was a time of incredible turmoil in the history of our country, as World War II had just begun. My aunt dropped out of college two months before graduation to get married and move to California. As soon as they arrived, her new husband was sent overseas to serve in the war, and she became Rosie the Riveter, working in a nearby defense plant. A stranger alone in a strange place, the stress was evidently too much. She developed rheumatoid arthritis. It was a lifelong struggle to live a normal life, but she perservered through work and college, earning a Ph.D. degree, despite enormous pain and depending at times on a wheelchair. I also have other relatives with arthritis. I have witnessed most personally the impact that arthritis has on one's everyday life. A part of me has lived in fear of this disease for most of my life.

At the age of 12 I had a swollen, inflamed, extremely painful knee. This lasted for about nine months, and no one was able to diagnose the problem. I must presume it was arthritis. Since my early twenties I have taken ibuprofen (Motrin or Advil) every day. If I don't take this medication for three consecutive days, my joints become extremely stiff and painful. So I take the medication and continue on my way. I have had joints injected with cortisone a dozen times in my adult life because of bursitis or tendinitis. The latest injection was for a painful hip, which was preventing me from exercising or climbing stairs.

When my youngest child, Elizabeth, was diagnosed at the age of 11 with juvenile rheumatoid arthritis, I had an impossible time accepting the fact. In our outrage at this injustice to the youngest member of the family, we waged a six-year battle with all the determination General Patton must have exerted to save Europe. Within three months of diagnosis my daughter had some 46 joints inflamed or swollen. At times she could not get out of bed. At times she could not stand for us to touch her. We were fortunate to have the best possible medical care. Bright, caring, compassionate people. People who encouraged her to fight the disease every step of the way. They guided us along the path, but we had to choose the right path. And, of course, all the people who loved Elizabeth contributed their strength to her battle through their love, concern, and desire to share her pain and overcome this disease. It felt as though we were "wrestling with the angel," and indeed it changed our lives.

If you have one of the many forms of arthritis and you are reading these lines, I presume you are not passively accepting that you *have* arthritis, or worse yet, that you are arthritic. That is the best news you could give me. I cannot tell you more emphatically that from my grandmother to my daughter, and many, many people in between, the victors in this battle, although they may have had every single joint in their bodies involved with arthritis, are those who *never let arthritis affect their hearts, their brains, or their spirits!*

From my personal experience, the battle against arthritis has to be a multifaceted approach. It requires many caring people but begins with ourselves. Healing begins within your own psyche by acknowledging the arthritis and learning to live the very best life you can until a cure is found for this disease. The people I have known with arthritis who have been most successful in life have shared a very similar pattern regardless of the severity of their arthritis. Although they may acknowledge the fact of the disease, I can assure you that they are not in the least accepting of the situation. As a matter of fact, the survivors seem to be among the most cantankerous! And at the risk of contradicting myself, another notable trait among survivors seems to be a well-developed sense of humor.

These people also know they need help, and they go about finding the very best help they can. They are extremely diligent. They take control and decide that arthritis will not dictate the direction of their lives. They might have to accommodate this mean intruder, but they do not let it choose which path they take.

One of the "pathfinders" who helped my daughter was Earl J. Brewer, Jr., M.D. With 30 years of experience in the field of rheumatology, he was instrumental in helping us choose the best possible medical care for her. Earl has a world of knowledge, and he is able to impart that knowledge in a no-nonsense manner. Today he remains a wonderful friend and collaborator. We have fought many battles together and shared many happy victories. I have observed Earl in many difficult situations, but probably my most overriding observation would be his compassion. He cares. He allows himself to care.

A Note from Earl

Let me address readers here as well by agreeing with everything Kathy has written above. The main lesson that I've learned in more than 30 years of caring for people with arthritis is that attitude and achievement are unrelated to how much pain and joint injury you have. While there are many people I know, let me mention one good example: Virgil Jones, assistant vice president in charge of statistical services of the Federal Reserve Bank of Kansas City. He has arthritis in virtually every joint of his body and needs assistance in many daily activities, yet he continues to travel the country by plane and car. As he says, "I don't have visions of grandeur. I know I can't be just like others, just Virg Jones contributing in some meaningful way to the people who cross my path and to the part of the world I touch. And that's why it is my perspective that 'the best I can be' isn't necessarily dependent on the physical limitations imposed by my arthritis."

An inspiring way to take charge of your destiny is exemplified by the president and chief operating officer of a Fortune 500 company, although she does not have arthritis. She always wears a bumblebee pin given to her by her mother years ago. "I finally asked her, 'Mom, I know you like this bee, but what does this mean?' She told me that aerodynamicists say that bumblebees shouldn't be able to fly, but no one told the bees, so they fly anyway. Now, whenever I get into a rough situation, or when I feel something is going to be particularly difficult, I look at the pin or touch it."

A major goal of this book is to point the way toward taking charge of your arthritis, living life to the fullest, and making your contribution.

A Note from Both

In writing this book we hope to share some of the knowledge we have learned. The most important message we have for anyone with arthritis is to *take control!* No one will care about your welfare more than you do. It is *your* life! As we Texans say, "Take the bull by the horns!"

The key to living successfully with arthritis is a four-step program, which we illustrate in this book. You need to understand the type of arthritis you have and what you should expect regarding the symptoms, prognosis, medications, and treatments. In Part 1 of this book, "Understanding Your Situation," we will therefore examine the many kinds of arthritis and their traditional therapies.

We have heard many people ask, "Why should I go to a doctor? They can't help me," or "Why should I try this new medication? It's like all the others. It won't help." With attitudes like these God Himself couldn't improve their situations. Healing has to begin within ourselves. A positive outlook is surely the best weapon in the medical arsenal.

Part 2, "Building a Team," addresses the importance of having a diverse team of experts on your side, and taking advantage of the variety of resources available to those with arthritis. In 1988, a team of researchers reported in *Arthritis & Rheumatism* that the damage they observed in a person's joints could not, by itself, explain the pain and difficulty that person experiences. They reported that attitude and emotions may have an even greater effect on the perception of pain. You *will* need help. Ideally people with arthritis should be treated by physicians trained in the field of rheumatology. Since there are some 37,000,000 people with arthritis and only 4,500 rheumatologists, you can calculate that there is an impossible number of patients for each doctor. Help will come in many forms, however, from your regular doctor to a rheumatologist, an internist, a psychologist, a physical therapist, an acupuncturist, and a host of others. And there are many "treatments" that at best don't help at all, and some that are downright dangerous. It is estimated that people are spending some eight billion dollars annually on these worthless or possibly hazardous treatments. We will examine those as well.

Your mission, should you decide to accept it, is to thoroughly educate yourself about your disease and all the possible treatments in order to choose the very best path for your life. The good news is that even though we can't alter the condition of our joints, we can certainly take charge of our own care. There are resources to help us in our search to improve our mental outlook—psychotherapy, self-hypnosis, positive imagery, relaxation techniques, biofeedback, and support groups, to mention a few. These in combination with proper medical care, good nutrition, and adequate exercise and rest should help you gain better control of your arthritis and your life.

Just how do you keep your life together? In Part 3, "Taking Care of Yourself," we will explore how to handle diet, exercise, rest, stress relief, and your emotional life. Your sexual needs will not change simply because you have arthritis. Communication between you and your partner becomes extremely important. Be open and be honest in assessing your need for affection. You have to care for yourself!

This section will also cover assistive devices, equipment that makes everyday activities easier for arthritics. You have to get out of bed, you have to comb your hair, you have to open a container of some kind for almost everything, and you have to perform whatever your life work is. It may be taking care of your home and family or it may be managing a large corporation, but whatever your work is, it is important to you. Taking care of yourself will enable you to do what you want.

If you have arthritis, each day brings special challenges. Depending on your stage of life, you may have to deal with the educational system, or you may have an employer who needs to be made aware of the effect arthritis has on your ability to do your job, or you may be facing the question of whether to have a child. If your arthritis is seriously damaging your joints, you will need to assess the possibility of having joint replacement surgery. In Part 4, "Paying Attention to Your Special Issues," we will address these and other issues that impact on people with arthritis.

Don't let arthritis become the focus of your life. Keep your eye on the goal—to live a happy, productive life.

Part One

UNDERSTANDING

YOUR

SITUATION

She beamed a smile across the room as I entered the premature nursery, her face barely visible over the incubator. Her eyes were framed by tortoise-shell glasses that slipped halfway down her nose, and her face was deeply lined with wrinkles from decades of smiles. Her starched white nurse's cap, as always, was in perfect place. She was gently lifting a small baby no longer than a submarine sandwich.

Looking a little closer, I saw her swollen fingers and wrists and caught her wincing a little as her wrist moved faster than she intended. This was Mrs. Potter, supervisor of the Halbouty Premature Nursery at St. Luke's Hospital in Houston, Texas, for at least 20 years. Her rheumatoid arthritis was so severe that several operations were necessary over a period of many years. Yet she rarely missed a day of work. Her pain some days almost brought tears to *my* eyes, but not hers.

You see, Mrs. Potter not only learned to live with arthritis, she was a better person because of it. She took control of her life and was determined to make her contribution. Mrs. Potter truly understood that there are challenges in life rather than problems, and that attitude is the determining factor, not how much she hurt.

During my 30 years of caring for people with arthritis, the two most important requests of patients and parents were for help in understanding what was wrong with their bodies and what could be done to lead as normal a life as possible. Many times I couldn't tell them the precise name for the pain in their joints, muscles, or tendons, but my understanding of what was going on within themselves and what they might expect gave them a starting point for moving on with their lives.

The old saying that we all are "hatched, matched, and dispatched" leaves out the essence of life as we would like to live it. Helping you live a better and fuller life *with* your arthritis rather than *in spite of* your arthritis is the goal. How you function and how you feel are far more important than telling you the precise name of a disease. After all, there are more than 100 types of arthritis, not to mention hundreds of variations of muscle and joint pain.

You may even be in the situation of not having a name for the pain, swelling, or tenderness you are feeling. Do not despair; most of us are in the same boat. We'll show you that while you are hurting a lot, you're not going to end up crippled. Also, there are many things you can do to live a better, happier, and fuller life.

Let's examine some terms first. *Rheumatism* is just a blanket term for a multitude of problems relating to joints or the muscles, tendons, and soft tissues that surround them. *Arthritis* means the swelling of a joint or the pain and tenderness that accompany limited motion. One tricky term is *arthralgia*. This "junior" arthritis means *pain only* and is limited to joints with no swelling or limited motion.

Doctors have precise ways to pinpoint different kinds of joint and muscle problems, so here are a few ground rules to help you understand. A term ending in *-itis* means that the part of the body indicated in the first part of the word is inflamed or has *inflammation*. *Arthron* is the Greek word for "joint," so *arthritis* (arthr- = joint + -itis) is inflammation of a joint such as the knee. *Inflammation* of a joint means that it is swollen, tender, warm to the touch, or red. This is the reaction of a joint such as the knee or wrist to being attacked by a germ, a foreign body such as a needle accidentally stuck into the joint, or an immune insult such as penicillin sensitivity, causing serum sickness and arthritis. The main *-itis* diseases we'll discuss are *rheumatoid arthritis* and *ankylosing spondylitis* (arthritis of the spine), but remember, there are at least a hundred more.

When you see *-osis* at the end of a word, it means an abnormal general condition that is not an inflammation. Thus, *osteoporosis* refers to an abnormal condition involving loss of calcium in the bone. Osteoporosis is a potentially serious problem among post-menopausal women because the loss of calcium weakens the bones and can cause fractures. We'll discuss ways to control osteoporosis in chapter 5.

Lastly, there is *osteoarthrosis,* or *osteoarthritis* (OA). Many people call it "old folks' arthritis" or degenerative joint disease, but it can happen to younger folks too. Both terms mean an abnormal general condition that produces degeneration of the bone *(osteo-)* or joint *(arthr-)* and generally occurs in people as they get older. OA also occurs secondary to injury from diseases such as rheumatoid arthritis or infections.

Studies of the progress of rheumatism (rather than the causes) show again and again that your ability to function in life is more useful to you and your doctor than expensive lab tests and X rays. In other words, *how you feel is how you are.*

Drs. Leigh Callahan and Ted Pincus at Vanderbilt School of

Medicine in Nashville have devoted years to studying hundreds of patients with many different kinds of arthritis, and they conclude that the best way to tell how you and your arthritis are progressing is by how well you function and what you can do. This doesn't mean that X rays and lab tests are not important; they are, but living well and healthily (and following the advice we provide in this book) will help you live a fuller and happier life more than the results of any test ever devised will.

Most of us having joint or muscle pains have no earthly idea why we are hurting, and if it doesn't last too long, we really don't care. But when the pain doesn't go away, we need to get serious about it. If you are at the stage where you are serious about your struggle and have found the answer with your doctor, then you're in good shape to move forward with your diagnosis for a better understanding of your situation.

1

Rheumatoid Arthritis

Driving to work with the windshield wipers beating a monotonous rhythm as they swished the rain from her field of vision, Charlotte rubbed her stiffened fingers and stretched them to get them moving. She squeezed her calf muscles, winced, and rolled her ankle to try to get comfortable, thinking to herself, *I don't know what idiot said that life begins at 40. Give me a break.*

By midmorning, Charlotte was already bone tired and snapped at her secretary when she accidentally interrupted Charlotte on the phone. As she stood up, her muscles just couldn't seem to get it together and were stiff until she started moving.

Two months later, after the playing first set of tennis at the Forest Club, Charlotte had to rest at the gazebo. She noticed that her knees were warm, swollen, and tender. Her friend Ria sat on the bench beside her and said, "Charlotte, you need to get your act together and go to the doctor to find out what's wrong. You're no fun anymore, and you move around like an old woman."

What Rheumatoid Arthritis Is

Rheumatoid arthritis (RA) is an *active, inflammatory, peripheral, symmetrical arthritis* afflicting three women for every man. Now let's break down this medical jargon. *Active* means that RA is an ongoing process lasting for years. In general parlance, *inflammatory* means fiery or provocative, but here it means swelling, redness, tenderness, and pain in your joints. *Peripheral* tells us that RA involves mainly the joints of the arms and legs, in particular the fingers and wrists. *Symmetrical* is the key in distinguishing it from other kinds of arthritis. RA usually involves the same joints on both sides of the body: the knees, the wrists, or the joints of the fingers, for example. Add to this definition *stiffness* of joints after inactivity and the requirement that arthritis last six weeks or longer in the same joints, and we have the official American College of Rheumatology definition for *rheumatoid arthritis*.

RA affects mainly women in their forties, but it can also occur in children and in seniors over 65 years of age. It is an equal opportunity condition, affecting rich and poor alike. One to three million Americans have RA. Arthritis occurs more than half of the time in the fingers, wrists, shoulders, knees, and ankles. Besides pain in the joints, it also causes trouble in other parts of the body, although involvement of the upper spine or lower sacroiliac joints is unusual.

Recognizing the Symptoms

The vignette about Charlotte, who experienced an onset of fatigue, irritability, inactivity stiffness, muscle pain, and symmetrical joint swelling, pain, warmth, and tenderness, illustrates the most common startup of this often capricious and potentially disruptive disease But while RA most often starts insidiously like Charlotte's arthritis did, for some people it strikes like a sledgehammer, hitting in one day and encompassing not only arthritis but fever, lumps under the skin (called rheumatoid nodules), muscle weakness, and loss of joint motion.

One of the most common symptoms of RA is fatigue. The pain of joint and muscle involvement is reason enough for fatigue, but even beyond that, people with RA are bone tired after just a few hours in the morning. Inability to sleep properly is common and contributes to this fatigue. Indeed, fatigue is one of the most important obstacles challenging you in taking control of your body and life.

Morning stiffness or inactive stiffness is also a prominent feature of RA. When it first happens to you, it's a little frightening. If you've been sitting for a while, standing up is suddenly difficult. There is a *gelling* of your muscles and joints, although this is not due only to pain. It may disappear after you move your muscles for a minute or two, but for some people it can last for many hours. Sometimes trying to get out of bed in the morning is impossible because of your morning stiffness.

You may have already found that your stiffness and pain are worse when the weather changes seasonally or even daily. In some people it is just before or just after the change! You become the weather person for the family. This is not a piece of foolishness; it is true. Studies in climate chambers show that a sudden drop in the barometric pressure or a sudden rise in the humidity does produce increased stiffness and pain in many people with arthritis. It is not specific to RA because it occurs in many people with old injuries to joints.

Another prominent feature of RA is the *rheumatoid nodule.* These are painless lumps you can feel under your skin. They occur on the bony part of the forearms, around the ankles, or even the pulp of the fingers. Some doctors think they are lumps of inflammation around small blood vessels. These lumps rarely cause problems and usually last only a few months. The nodules can occur in other rheumatic diseases as well.

Inflammation is another symptom and can lead to injury to the joints. However, months and even years can pass before sufficient injury to the joints shows up in X rays. Your doctor may wish to take X rays anyway for two reasons: to rule out injury or other diseases, and to take a baseline X ray for later comparison. So don't feel put upon; it's probably a good idea.

More than the joints are involved in RA. Inflammation of the tendons, muscles, and tissues around the joints also causes trouble by reducing your life-style and functioning due to pain. Injury to these tissues also can cause deformity and problems with joint motion and strength. To help you understand the jargon, remember the *-itis* and *–algia* terms. Inflammation of a muscle is *myositis*, and pain in a muscle is *myalgia*. Inflammation of the tendons is *tendinitis*, and pain in a tendon is *tenalgia*, but for some reason no one uses it. The soft tissues around the joints can be affected by *fibrositis*.

Rarely, RA afflicts the large organs of the body such as the lungs, liver, kidney, arteries, and heart. The skin can also develop a variety of rashes and discolorations that are not serious.

We need to spend a little time talking about your inflamed and swollen joints. Feel your knee or fingers that are swollen. The first thing you notice is that they are tender to the touch. They are also probably a little warm, but not red. Notice how thick and boggy they feel compared to your other joints that are not swollen. This thickness is inflammation of the *joint capsule,* or covering of the joint. You may feel a squishy sensation when you push on the joint. This is the fluid that is inside the joint capsule. The fluid can cause pressure on the cartilage that covers the ends of the bone. This pressure, plus the inflammatory cells and chemicals in the fluid can cause injury to the *cartilage* and even to the *bone*. As these changes occur, the *muscles* and *tendons* around the joint become weak from pain and less frequent use, resulting in loss of motion and contractures. It is wise to pay close attention to this problem and enter into an aggressive treatment program if you want to keep functioning the way you expect.

The *rheumatoid factor* (RF) is another feature of RA. It is an *auto-antibody* (*auto* = the human body; + *antibody* = the immune system of the body fighting off an outside antigen). The RF test is important because at least 8 out of 10 people with RA test positive for RF. However, RF also occurs with other conditions and diseases and is therefore not completely indicative in a diagnosis. Paradoxically, some experts think it causes injury to the joints, while others believe it is how the body fights off RA. Either way, it makes little difference to most people. If you are RF positive and have chronic arthritis, the chances are overwhelming that you have RA.

Other laboratory blood tests conducted on people with RA often reveal a mild anemia. One test, called the *sed rate,* or *erythrocyte sedimentation rate,* is elevated in inflammatory diseases and is used by your doctor as a guide to monitoring the activity of your disease. You will also hear of a test called the *ANA,* or *antinuclear antibody test.* This test is positive in people with lupus, another rheumatic disease usually affecting young women, but 1 out of 10 people with RA also have positive ANA. The level of the positive test is much lower than that seen in people with lupus.

Knowing the Patterns

RA is usually active for six to eight years and then levels off. However, if you still have arthritis two years after onset, the chances are that you're going to have continuing joint problems, and you will need to follow a program of care for yourself such as the one suggested in this book.

Some people, however, are more lucky. Your chances are about

1 in 5 that you will have RF negative arthritis and, therefore, your course of illness will be milder. You may also have intermittent remissions of swelling lasting more than one year, and your periods of inactive arthritis may be longer than those in which your arthritis is active.

Several rheumatologists have observed that a small group of patients who have onset of RA after age 60 also have a milder course of illness with more remissions than do younger patients with RA. Others note that perhaps 1 in 10 RA patients have remissions after the first bout but no further trouble afterward.

Investigating the Causes

In truth, no one knows the causes of RA. However, it is especially important to know that *you* did not *cause* your rheumatoid arthritis. Neither your life–style nor anything you might have taken has induced it. Several rheumatologists were asked to comment on this. Their answers were remarkably similar. Each tells his or her patients that they must not feel guilty, that they somehow did something wrong and developed RA.

Many doctors and scientists believe there is a genetic predisposition to RA that, when triggered, causes the onset of the disease. Seven out of 10 people with RA are found to have a particular inherited chemical marker *(antigen)* on the surface of almost all of their cells. By comparison, fewer than 3 out of 10 nonafflicted people have this antigen, which seems to indicate some kind of correlation. In addition there are many families like Kathy's who have had several generations with RA. There are so many associated factors that it is difficult to make any sense of it. The truth is that like life itself, there are undoubtedly several factors that must be present before RA occurs.

One of the keys is the *immunogenetics* of RA. When attacked, the immune system of the body somehow turns on itself and produces chronic inflammation of the joints and other tissues. If you get a thorn or a large splinter under your skin, the skin around the area becomes red, then warm and swollen. Fluid and pus form as the body attempts to get rid of the foreign body. Many chemical and immune reactions are produced by the cells of the body to make this happen. The body reacts pretty much the same way in trying to get rid of any foreign body, and the immune system of the body manufactures antibodies to help get rid of them. Germs causing infection are attacked in the same way. As explained earlier, in rheumatoid arthritis the body creates autoantibodies that attack the joints, causing redness and swelling in the lining of the joints. Fluid and pus cells pour into the joint space. Again, your system is trying to get rid of a foreign body, only in the case of RA we can't seem to find out what the foreign body is.

Many associated factors and events also occur at the onset of RA that are important to understand. The first is that RA occurs in women three times as often as in men. Even more startling is that when women with RA become pregnant, not only do they get better, but the disease often goes away completely. It is astounding to see a young, fatigued woman with swollen, stiff, and painful fingers and joints, suddenly blossom into a smiling, happy person able to move normally a month or so after becoming pregnant. Unfortunately, six weeks or so after her baby is delivered, the arthritis returns, sometimes with a vengeance.

Second, RA is associated with various infections at the onset of illness. Because it is natural to assume that if something happens just before or at the same time that RA begins, the number of factors that are said to cause it are legion. Almost every infection you can imagine has been implicated—strep throat, mononucleosis, many other viruses, and other micro-organisms. But it is increasingly clear that many infections can trigger the onset of RA.

However, it also appears that severe stress plays a role. The death of a family member, a divorce or separation, loss of a job, or a significant injury can all trigger the onset of RA. One teenage patient of mine experienced the onset of his arthritis when he fell off the back of a moving truck. Miraculously he didn't break any legs, but from that moment on he had serious and crippling arthritis.

Cold, wet weather can also trigger RA in those who are genetically predisposed. Rheumatologists generally claim that about two-thirds of people with RA begin their disease in the winter, and infections are certainly more common in the winter.

Determining the Prognosis

Your attitude toward life, RA, and how you handle both have more to do with your prognosis and outlook than all of the facts we are about to discuss. Taking control of your destiny, remaining active, and exercising will have a greater effect on how well you function than most any therapy.

RA is a burn-in, burn-out disease. With active arthritis, the swelling, pain, and tenderness progresses in starts and stops for about six to eight years. You'll have bad days, weeks, or months. You'll have days where the stiffness and pain make you want to stay in bed, and other days when you can jump out of bed without any problems.

In the worst-case scenario, you may experience a leveling off after a few years, just when you think it will never end. The swelling goes away, and you forget how long it's been since bad weather laid you low. You are, however, left with whatever damage and injury RA did to your joints during those first years. Much of this damage is due to osteoarthritis and damage to cartilage secondary to RA. You may have difficulty picking up socks or twisting off bottle caps. It may also be tough to walk.

If you are in this category, the active exercise program we encourage you to follow, and other aggressive treatments of your RA, may enable you to carry out the normal activities of life. Your attitude must not allow you to give up.

If you are thinking, *What does all that mean between the lines?* it means that some people with RA will inevitably have much injury to many joints, muscles, and tendons. The weakness and pain from these deformities will restrict their activities more than they would like. Having said that, however, let us add that how you function depends on how you feel, and it really doesn't make any difference what your X rays look like or what the RF test result is. You may need to consider surgery and joint replacements, which we'll discuss in chapter 18. Overall, even if you have a case of arthritis, there's a lot you can do to change your situation. RA rarely causes trouble in other parts of the body, such as the blood vessels, lungs, liver, heart, and kidneys. Insurance companies may have a fit over a slightly increased mortality in RA, but the reality is that you should not lose any sleep over it.

But that's the worst-case outlook. Let's now talk about the best-case scenario for you. One in 4 or 5 people with RA will have an initial bout of arthritis but within two years will be free of arthritis and have no more trouble. People in this group are more likely to be RF negative.

A Course of Treatment

Let's dispose of two myths about the treatment of arthritis. Both are blatantly wrong.

MYTH 1: *There's nothing you can do about arthritis, so why bother?*
Over the past 20 years, most of the rheumatologists I know recog-

nize that we now see few long-term RA invalids. Things have changed since more aggressive treatments came about, whereas earlier many people with RA ended up in bed full-time.

Why? One principal reason is the widespread use of non-steroidal anti-inflammatory drugs (NSAIDs) and other medicines (which we'll talk about in chapter 10) that can reduce pain enough to allow RA sufferers to function better in life. They also sufficiently reduce the inflammation of the disease in the joints to allow greater mobility.

MYTH 2: *Staying in bed will save my joints from injury.*
On the contrary, keeping active and living life to its fullest is the key to doing well. This does not mean *going to bed and staying there.* We now know that staying in bed full-time results in weaker, smaller muscles as well as the loss of calcium from the bones, which can lead to fractures and other problems. The joints get stiff and quit moving. For a long time doctors thought that as folks get older they lose muscle mass and get fatter and certainly weaker. But an interesting study done with senior citizens over age 70 contradicted that view. The participants in that study exercised in a class for about 20 minutes three times a week doing aerobics and other movement exercises, while a control group did what they usually did—watch TV or play bingo. In six months the exercise group was not only more agile but gained over 10 percent in muscle strength and mass and lost over 10 percent in body fat. So much for casting medical facts in stone. We'll discuss exercise further in chapter 13.

In short, the cornerstone of your treatment program is to function as normally as possible. Take charge of your RA and intelligently use and coordinate the services of a wide variety of people. Get in partnership with your doctor—preferably a rheumatologist—who will be a partner with you in planning the best life-style program for you. You want to be as active as possible, although you do need to balance active exercise with rest. Fatigue is a big problem early in the disease. Medications can reduce the *synovitis,* or inflammation of the joints, as well as reduce your pain. These two actions allow you not only to get around but to actively exercise and keep up your strength. Chapter 11 will focus on these medications.

I promised you earlier that we would help with your stiffness, and we'll do it in detail in Parts 2 and 3, but for now you should know that NSAIDs sometimes do the trick. Other tricks that help include sleeping in a waterbed or taking warm baths in the early morning. Getting up and moving around every once in a while sometimes cuts stiffness off at the pass. In addition, proper nutrition is essential. Unless you are taking in enough food and the proper foods, you will only get weaker. There are no special diets that cure arthritis. We'll provide you with ground rules about diet in chapter 14.

You may need splints at times to keep joints such as the wrist from drifting at an awkward angle. There is catalog after catalog of assistive devices that will make life easier if you have weakness and pain in your hands, for instance. My favorite is a special bottle-cap opener—it's so handy that I use it, and I don't even have arthritis. We'll clue you in on this and more in chapter 16. Finally, just in case you are in that group who has serious injury to hips, knees, or other joints, orthopedists have done a spectacular job in returning bedridden RA sufferers to pain-free, near-normal walking with joint replacements.

Now that you know the ground rules, move forward on the path to taking charge and making life with RA more enjoyable for you.

2

Osteoarthritis

One day at the Forest Club I arrived late for my tennis game and found that I had left my size 13B Reeboks at home. My solution was to play in socks. I started out well enough on the limestone-and-clay court, but after a set of running and skidding in the dirt, the heels and balls of my feet cried for mercy. I had to stop for the day, and my poor feet were swollen and painful for the next week. I thought that since our ancestors spent their days barefoot, I could do without the air cushion of my $50 tennis shoes for a couple of hours. Not true.

This was my personal lesson in the value of a shock absorber or cushion for the feet, especially my 64-year-old feet. The body understands this need too, and nearly every joint of our bodies has a cushion or shock absorber for all that bouncing and bounding about that we do daily. If we didn't, the bones of the knee, the ankle, the elbow, and every other joint would grind each other to pieces. This shock absorber is called *cartilage*. (Animals have it too, of course, and we know it as *gristle*.) It covers the ends of the bones and is full of water and elastic tissue that gives so well when you jump on it that you could patent it for a waterbed if you could figure out how to do so. Every time you jump up and down, the pressure exerted on your hips or knees is four to eight times your weight, and the only way for the body to tolerate this load is for the cartilage to absorb the enormous pressure by squeezing together like a sponge and then rebounding to its original shape. It does this over and over again for your entire life.

Like everything else in our bodies, however, cartilage sooner or later wears out or is injured. For instance, a ring of cartilage with fluid in the middle is located between each of the backbones as a cushion for the spinal column. Sometimes, the ring of cartilage is torn and the fluid leaks out. This is called a ruptured disc and it is extremely painful.

What Is Osteoarthritis?

There are many reasons why cartilage injury occurs, but when it does, the injury progresses to loss of this protective shock absorber. Bone rubs against bone, causing osteoarthritis. OA is a disease of the cartilage and leads to injury of the joint. It is not due simply to wear and tear or old age. Some physicians think of it as the end result of any injury to a joint. Osteoarthritis is split into *idiopathic* or *primary* OA. We have no explanation as to where it comes from or what causes it. *Secondary* OA means that a specific joint injury (such as a football injury or an infection) or other joint disease (such as RA) occurred. Other causes of secondary OA are congenital defects of the joint, and metabolic disorders (such as gout) causing injury to the cartilage and joint.

OA is not like RA in that it does not affect symmetrical parts of the body. Three main areas of the body are affected most often:

1. *Fingers*: Heberden's nodes look like the bumps you got on the end of your index finger from holding your pencil so tightly in elementary school, except these can develop on any finger and on both sides of the nail. Heberden's nodes are made of cartilage and bone. Most of the time they are painless and only cause cosmetic problems. However, sometimes they develop suddenly and are painful and tender. The joint at the end of the finger can also be swollen, red, and tender. Called *nodal* OA, this form occurs in women older than 45 years by a ratio of 10:1 over men. It is thought to be hereditary and dominant.

2. *Hip and knee*: OA of weight-bearing joints occurs more frequently in men and may be due to the types of heavy physical work done more often by men. The abuse in these joints can at times be severe enough to require joint replacement.

3. *Spine:* The joints connecting the upper parts of the spine together and the joints of the spine itself can develop OA. The chief problem in the spine is when the bony spurs impinge on the nerves, causing pain or loss of function.

Osteoathritis afflicts as many as 40 million people in the country. A national health survey showed that it can begin as early as the second decade of life, and by the fifth decade 90 percent of us have at least some visible changes in our cartilage, although 1 in 5 of us actually has moderate or severe disease due to OA. It is another equal opportunity condition, with men generally affected as often as women overall. However, there are subsets of OA in which women and men differ in frequency and type. Women have OA of the fingers more often, while men have OA of the knees and hips more often. Some doctors believe that the lifestyles of both men and women account for the differences. However, women with nodal OA in the fingers are thought to have an autosomal, sex-influenced, dominant gene directly related to their OA.

Where you live seems to be a factor. The warmer the climate, the worse it is. Eskimos and other ethnic groups living in cold environments have less OA. Weight also has an effect: OA of the knees is worse in obese people, although part of this problem may be a sedentary life-style or a diet of saturated fats. Since four to eight times of your body weight presses on your knees when you are jumping or climbing stairs, it only makes sense that every pound of extra fat adds four to eight pounds more stress on the knees and hips.

Another category of people prone to OA are hypermobiles, such as girls who can bend their ankles around their necks or do a split with one leg straight in front and one in back, or kids who can bend their thumbs back to touch their forearms. This hypermobility is useful for ballet, gymnastics, or diving, but such misuse and overuse can cause injury to the joints and bring on OA earlier than in other folks. My wife and I have a hypermobile daughter who was a national and collegiate diver for 10 years, but now, in her mid-twenties, she has chronic back pain.

Some activities of life also seem to cause more OA in certain parts of the body. I mention this to remind you that you need to pay attention to the proper use of joints. People engaged in heavy lifting occupations such as mining have a lot more OA of the knees and hips than do office workers. Women employed in weaving jobs often develop OA in their favored hand.

People frequently ask me, "Then why do you push me to do all that exercise?" The primary reason is that research has shown that runners have little evidence of injury to the cartilage of the joint, so running is actually good exercise for many people. *However*, if your joints swell after jogging or walking, listen to what your body is telling you, and exercise some other way.

Recognizing the Symptoms

Ironically, only about a third of people whose X rays show they have OA ever have much pain or other symptoms. But if you are one of them, here's what to look for. Early on, aching pain in your fingers or knee, for example, will occur after exercise but will go away after you rest a bit. The painful joints may be stiff only a few minutes at a time and usually aren't warm or swollen, but over a period of months or even years the occasional pain may progress to continual pain after even minimal use and motion. You'll know it's really bad when the pain wakes you up at night or keeps you from sleeping. (This is where a waterbed comes in handy; we'll address this in chapter 15.)

Eventually, as the cartilage is worn away more until bone crunches on bone, a grating feeling or sound can be felt or heard when the joint is moved. This is called *crepitus*. You may experience limitation of joint motion and pain upon motion. There will also be localized tenderness where the joint is touched. At this point there may be enough injury to the joint and the cartilage that secondary synovitis ensues, causing a disconcerting warmth and swelling to the joint, known as *erosive* inflammatory osteoarthritis.

You may also develop *osteophytes,* which are outpouchings of bone at the edges of joints such as the knee and spine. Nerves that connect the spine to the muscles can be injured when lumps of bone, or osteophytes, form at the edge of the joints of the spine, and these osteophytes can squeeze the nerves, causing severe pain. These hard lumps can form on the edge of the knee, for instance; they can be tender and are also responsible for the bony enlargement in the fingers.

As OA progresses, loss of motion of a joint or joints becomes more and more of a possibility. Many internal changes are happening: an uneven surface of the joint can develop due to loss of cartilage on one side, with muscle spasms around the joint due to pain, a shortening of tendons and muscles, and osteophytes. In a few individuals, serious deformities of certain joints occur. Again, however, most people with OA do not experience such serious progressive crippling.

Laboratory tests for OA are a normal procedure but are not useful except to rule out other conditions. X rays can show the degree of injury to the cartilage and bone. Although the cartilage does not show up on X ray because it does not have any calcium salts, when cartilage is injured and the cushion is reduced in size, the joint space is reduced on X ray, allowing the doctor to determine the extent of injury. Unfortunately, these findings are not helpful early in the condition, since they can only be detected after significant loss has already occurred.

Investigating the Causes

As I have said, many factors seem to contribute to OA, with genetics, aging, trauma, and chemical changes in the body among the most important. Obesity or local inflammation of a joint also are closely associated. If OA is indeed the end result of any joint injury, nearly any possible cause may be valid. However, recent studies point to a genetic predisposition. In a few people OA appears in X rays as early as the teenage years. Aging is certainly a factor, and it may be true that in different people the cartilage simply wears out at different ages. Nothing is forever. We know that the appearance of OA is more frequent as we get older.

Trauma may be as important a cause as genetics and aging. We know that a blow to a joint from an athletic injury, for example, can produce pain and changes many years after the main injury occurred. Similarly, it can be argued that OA of the fingers is often due to a life of repeated-motion injury, as in women who work in weaving factories. We also know that impact injury is an important cause of damage to cartilage. This is probably why baseball, basketball, and diving injuries are so frequently associated with secondary OA.

The numerous chemical reactions of the body that control the metabolism of cartilage in the joint can misfire at any time and cause injury to the cartilage. For example, if the manufacture of new cartilage and elimination of old cartilage are altered when chemical enzyme digestion (chemicals that break down cartilage) goes awry, or when or an inflammatory disease begins, then OA can result.

Determining the Prognosis

Before beginning the task of writing this book, several people with long-standing arthritis were interviewed to find out what lessons they wanted to impart. The single universal lesson they learned was that *there is life during and after arthritis.* You must stay with the mainstream of life and take control of your arthritis rather than letting your arthritis control you. As mentioned before, the vast majority of people develop OA as they get older, but only about a fourth get worse in terms of increased pain, deformity, instability, and decreased function.

Can you do something about it if it happens to you? Yes, of course you can. OA need not continue to get worse and worse. In many people it progresses to a certain point and then remains the same. It is not true that if you have nodal OA of the fingers in your forties that you'll have a worsening of the disease in your sixties. The ultimate outlook of primary OA depends on where it is located and how bad it is. If you have OA in the fingers, unless you're a concert pianist or a heart surgeon, you can probably make do. However, if you have it in the legs, your hips and knees can become so painful or unstable that joint replacement is necessary; *but* at least you can do something about it.

Spinal OA is perhaps the worst because in a few people the osteophytes growing from the edges of the joints of the spine squeeze the nerves and cause pain and weakness in the arms or legs. Surgery may be needed to ream out the bone to relieve the pressure on the nerves. Don't cringe too much—this doesn't happen very often.

A Course of Treatment

In the interviews conducted with people with arthritis, virtually everyone said that the main thing they wanted to convey is that exercise is truly helpful, especially swimming. Dr. Rollie Moskowitz, a rheumatologist famous for his work with OA patients, offers this advice: "There are too many *don'ts* in life, but one *do* is to remain active and to exercise."

I therefore heartily recommend that you hook up with an exercise trainer at a YMCA or health club to plan a program for you. You don't necessarily have to be a member of a health club to hire a trainer, however. Many trainers work independently for a fee. Ask at the health club or YMCA for names. If you have access to a pool, use it, because the water's buoyancy protects your joints from impact injury. If you don't have access to a pool, use the equipment found in professional gyms such as exercise cycles and Stairmasters. Walking is great, but in my view it's a distant third to these other two forms of exercise. (For details about exercise tools and equipment, see chapter 13.) Therapeutic exercises for specific joints such as your fingers should be done under the guidance of your doctor and physical therapist at a clinic or hospital. If you don't get the right information there, ask your exercise trainer.

A proper life-style is vital. The way to feel better and be healthier is to get the right amount of rest, eat the right foods in the right amounts, and lay off those three-martini lunches or dinners. Smoking is a guaranteed way to leave this life earlier than you plan. Be sure you're a member of the flock that thinks Coke is only a soft drink and nothing more.

There are also many assistive devices to help you partake in the joys of daily life. Even if OA causes you to have limited motion and strength, there are still lots of ways to do what you want to do. There are devices that will open not only cans and bottles, but also car doors and kitchen doors. Thanks to handy remote controls that turn on and off everything from the TV to the microwave to the garage door, it's really shaping up to be a good era for people with limitations due to arthritis. With the new disability laws, curbs, steps, and stores are going to be more arthritis friendly. Probably the most helpful device is the simplest and oldest—the walking cane. If you use one, be sure that it's the right length. The salesman at the store can measure that for you. It's also good to take advantage of stores that offer grocery delivery services to people who have trouble getting out. (For more information, see chapter 16.)

You can also obtain pain relief by taking acetaminophen or Tylenol-like drugs, which are recommended by many rheumatologists. However, inflammatory arthritis is probably more common than everyone lets on, and for this reason the nonsteroidal anti-inflammatory drugs (NSAIDs) such as aspirin, Advil, and Naprosyn help relieve pain in or near joints not responsive to Tylenol as well as relieve the swelling of inflamed joints. Local injections of cortisone derivatives into selected joints are sometimes used to relieve painful, swollen joints temporarily. Sometimes it is difficult to know whether removing the fluid helps or if NSAIDS are better. In any event, we suggest you use injections sparingly. Chapter 10 provides more details about this and NSAIDs in general.

Finally, surgery is considered as a therapy for OA. It is seldom needed, but when recommended, joint replacements of hips and knees have been a godsend for people with OA and many other kinds of arthritis. The relief of pain and improvement of motion has renewed life for hundreds of thousands of people in the past 20 years. Chapter 18 will discuss surgery in greater detail.

3

Fibromyalgia

Fibrositis, Bursitis, Tendinitis, and Related Ailments

Penelope, sitting erect on the edge of her chair, nervously crossed one knee over the other while smoothing the material of her green linen suit. She looked directly at the doctor and said, "I know I'm probably being presumptuous, but you're the tenth doctor I've seen, and I really need some help." Rushing on, not giving her doctor a chance to interrupt, Penelope added, "My husband's about to give up on me; I'm in my late forties; I hurt, it seems like everywhere, at some time during the day. And another thing—I'm so stiff in the morning, and I'm so tired that I feel like I haven't even been to bed. Even worse, I just sit around the house and mope."

Smiling, Dr. Mary White held up her hands, to form a T for time out. She said, "Hey, slow down, you're with a friend now. You hurt. I believe you. Now let's figure out how to help you."

What Is Fibromyalgia?

Fibromyalgia evokes a fiery, mixed response among arthritis doctors wherever they may gather. Sensible, reserved, elder statesmen of medicine turn red in the face, ready to explode while impatiently waiting to blast or laud the believers and the nay-sayers.

The reason for the turmoil is that not every doctor recognizes fibromyalgia. I believe that fibromyalgia is a real entity, and so do many other rheumatologists; however, many extremely competent doctors believe it to be entirely emotional and cite a long list of personality traits, especially those related to depression, as the real culprits.

For the moment then, let's accept that it does exist and try to define it better. *Fibro-* (*fibrous,* for the soft tissues of the body under the skin, especially around the joints including tendons and ligaments), *my-* (*myo,* for muscle), and *-algia* (pain) mean pain in the supporting tissues of the body, such as tissues around the knee or muscles around the shoulder. People sometimes write about *fibrositis* and *fibromyalgia* in the same sentence, but the terms mean the same thing. It is important, though, to mention that there is a big difference between generalized fibromyalgia and local pain in tendons (tendinitis), bursa (bursitis), or muscles (myositis). These localized areas of pain or inflammation are either secondary to a disease such as rheumatoid arthritis or caused by misuse, overuse, or underuse.

Fibromyalgia happens mostly to women in their forties, lasts for years, and varies in severity on any given day. However, I have also encountered teenagers with *fibromyalgia* as well as people over 60. Also, the severity of fibromyalgia is inconsistent. On some days, a sufferer may be bursting with energy, while on other days fatigue, tender points of pain over fairly predictable parts of the body, and stiffness of muscles will ensue. Waking up in the morning still feeling tired after a night's sleep is also a common sign. Ironically, perhaps 20 percent of patients who visit an arthritis doctor have *fibromyalgia*, though not all doctors are willing to recognize this.

Recognizing the Symptoms

There is a four-symptom complex that should trigger a doctor to think of fibromyalgia. The first is *chronic, diffuse musculoskeletal pain*. This is the most important and essential symptom. The sufferer feels pain in the muscles; however, when the doctor begins to poke and punch here and there, the pain is triggered by tender points that are about an inch or so wide and make the fibromyalgic person jump with pain. These tender points are not on the skin but are produced when deep pressure is applied. The locations of these pressure-tender points are shown in Figure 1.

Why they are located in these spots is unknown, but it is amazing to me how reproducible the tender points are, not only in the same person but also in others with fibromyalgia. There are at least 8 of these points, and some doctors recognize 14 or more. Of course, not every person with *fibromyalgia* has all of the tender points, nor do they have them all of the time. Indeed, the pain is so variable on a day-to-day basis that many a doubting Thomas think the sufferer is seeking attention or faking. Doctors can also be skeptical because they cannot see any swelling or other usual indications of disease. Many doctors truly feel that if they can't see disease, it must be in the brain and not in the body. (Something that I still find difficult to grasp is that the brain can indicate the location of pain in the skin but lacks the ability to pinpoint pain in muscles and other deep tissues.) However, the cause of a tender point can easily be found. For instance, a tender point just below the inside of the elbow (Figure 1) can actually be traced to a muscle, where it arises from the head of the radius bone some distance

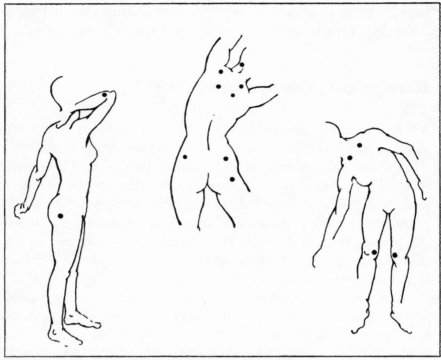

Figure 1: Locations of pressure-tender points

away. What seems to be superficial pain with no cause is actually *referred pain* from a deeper muscle or tendon that is having trouble. A more familiar example of referred pain is the referred pain of appendicitis to the right lower quadrant of the stomach. There is certainly no disease in the skin, but there's something wrong with the deeply hidden appendix. For this reason and others, I am not troubled over an inability to explain the lack of local disease at the tender points of fibromyalgia.

The second of the big four symptoms is *nonrejuvenating sleep*. This means that you wake up more tired than when you went to sleep the night before. Related to this is the third major finding, *fatigue*. These two symptoms usually cause more alteration in lifestyle than the pain does.

The fourth symptom is *stiffness of muscles* in the mornings, usually lasting a short time but occasionally lasting all day. While the stiffness doesn't seem to produce the "gelling" effect of RA stiffness, meaning that getting out of bed is not a problem in fibromyalgia, it is nevertheless troublesome and a sure symptom.

When these symptoms are taken together and last months and years, fibromyalgia is the probable diagnosis. Note that all four symptoms can vary in intensity and occur independently on any given day; thus, stiffness and fatigue may be worse one day, and pain may be worse on another day. Nevertheless, they all point to fibromyalgia.

Additionally, other prominent features include headaches and *paresthesia*. Paresthesia refers to a tingly, prickly sensation. For example, the skin over tender points around the knee, elbow, or upper back can be hypersensitive to a pin prick which will cause more pain than it should. This is similar to the referred pain of the right lower quadrant of the tummy when appendicitis occurs, and so this feature does not indicate some psychiatric problem but is entirely compatible with referred pain manifestations. The headaches are nonspecific, but look at Figure 1 again, and you can see that there are tender points in the neck at the base of the skull. At least some of the headaches may be related to these points.

As with most kinds of arthritis, stress and anxiety make fibromyalgia worse, as do flu, asthma, and any other illness. Some doctors believe that there is a presumed fibromyalgia personality (the overachieving, noncomplaining individual) and that the features of fibromyalgia are caused directly by preceding depression, anxiety, and stress. However, other doctors, including myself, believe as already discussed that depression, anxiety, and stress are the *result* of the features of fibromyalgia, not the cause.

Investigating the Causes

Given the above, what does cause fibromyalgia? The most sensible explanation is referred pain from muscle, fat, or fascia (the tough, soft tissue covering of muscles). Unfortunately, what causes the trouble in the muscles and other tissues is unknown. Examining the tissues fails to show disease as we know it. One idea is that the brain sends messages of pain to the body after chemical stimulation of nerve cells in the brain. This is called pain modulation or down regulation of endorphins. We know, for example, that rheumatic fever is caused by a hypersensitivity, usually to a strep infection of the throat. Some doctors believe that fibromyalgia is a similar reaction to an infection. Again, this is theory but it is certainly possible. Additionally, abnormalities of sleep patterns on electroencephalograms (EEGs) have been found in fibromyalgia sufferers, although the meaning is not known. Exposure to wet, bad weather certainly makes it worse or triggers it.

Determining the Prognosis

The good news is that people with fibromyalgia do not generally have serious long-term arthritis or crippling ailments. In other words, fibromyalgia is not the beginning of a serious rheumatic disease. You may hurt a lot or incur chronic fatigue, but you will not have to deal with joints that are damaged later. Many people who have RA, OA, or something similar may have secondary fibromyalgia, but the point is that they had RA first and fibromyalgia later, not the reverse. One puzzling aspect of the prognosis is that when women with fibromyalgia become pregnant, the symptoms can go away during the pregnancy, just as with RA.

A Course of Treatment

In general, though fibromyalgia waxes and wanes with the years, it stays and stays and stays. This is an important factor for you to understand because there are things you can do to get on with your life: *First, stop feeling sorry for yourself.* Take charge of your life and set goals. Start by getting out of bed, no matter how much it hurts. No matter how tired you are, you can begin doing something. *You must begin by building your endurance again.* Many folks respond that it's well and good to give a pep talk about getting on with life, and they agree that the pain is bearable. *But*—and this is a big *but*—being constantly tired is what prevents a semblance of normal activity. So what do you do? We recommend swimming every day with the AquaJogger as the best way to get started. This is a water buoyancy belt that fits around your waist and holds you up in the water. The belt costs about $50. There is also a video-cassette that outlines your workout in the water for about $20. The AquaJogger is really useful, especially if you use it regularly and consistently. On the first day, aquajog only a few minutes, then increase the time daily to build up your strength and endurance. You can order the AquaJogger by calling 1-800-922-9544. (For more information on using the AquaJogger, see pages 146–148.)

Next, ask friends, relatives, or even health professionals to *help you find a quality health club with first-rate and certified exercise trainers.* Have your trainer help you create an exercise program, and follow the program every day for half an hour or so. After you have a program, don't feel locked in with a trainer forever. Once you know the ropes, you can wing it on your own and limit paying the trainer to periodic sessions, since your health insurance probably won't cover it. File a claim for it anyway; some insurance companies understand the necessity for exercise treatment.

The fourth thing to do is to *make your sleep as comfortable as possible.* You may wish to consider a waterbed. Waterbeds have come a long way in design since the early days; they now have cylinders or tubes of thick vinyl about four inches wide running lengthwise, and you can make them as firm or soft as you want, anytime you want. They also have heaters for each side of the bed, and the cost is about half that of a quality mattress and springs. A 1989 Gallup poll among waterbed users and regular mattress users revealed that the waterbed won hands down in relieving back pain. Older people, in fact, are now the main buyers of waterbeds. You can rent one at some places to see how you like it. The purpose, of course, is to see whether you get more rest and wake up rejuvenated instead of nonrejuvenated.

Lastly, to counter pain, fatigue, and nonrejuvenating sleep, I don't recommend NSAIDs as your primary therapy. For whatever reason, the aspirins, the Advils, the Voltarens, and the Naprosyns don't really seem to work, nor do any of the other 15 or more NSAIDs on the market. Instead, you have to focus on exercise.

The tricyclic medicines, however, are useful for people with fibromyalgia. There are several medicines in the tricyclic group, but you can't take all of them. Ask your doctor about Elavil (amitriptyline) and Sinequan (doxepin); both have several actions and are principally used to help stressed people. They also have physiologic effects on the nervous system that may explain the improvement in fatigue and nonrejuvenating sleep that occurs in many people with fibromyalgia. The medicines are generally taken at night, but you must be supervised by your doctor.

In the long run, though, remember that the only person who can help is yourself. Plan an exercise program—preferably one with a pool—and start today. The later chapters will point the way in more detail.

4

Ankylosing Spondylitis

The mention of *ankylosing spondylitis* (AS) immediately brings to mind low back pain. The two are so intertwined that the most common complaint of people suffering from AS is back pain. Whereas for most people back pain lasts a few days or weeks due to misuse or overuse, with AS the pain lasts and lasts. Often it is not until after three months that you realize that AS has crept up on you.

What Is Ankylosing Spondylitis?

AS is a chronic inflammatory disease causing mainly arthritis of the spine. The term is broken down to mean *ankylosing* (fused, stiff, or rigid), *spondyl-* (spine), and *-itis* (inflammation). It was thought to be a part of RA for many years, but now we know that it is related but separate. AS is an ancient disease of human-kind and has been found even in Egyptian mummies. Some medical historical sleuths trace it back to some of our Darwinian cousins: monkeys, crocodiles, and horses.

As many as two million Americans have AS, but it occurs in men three or four times more often than in women as opposed to RA. AS is often a disease of young people beginning mostly in their twenties and thirties. There is a genetic marker on the cells of people with AS called HLA-B27, which establishes a genetic predisposition to AS and helps to explain why there is such a disparity in frequency of AS among races. The incidence of HLA-B27 varies from about 8 percent in Anglos in the United States to 1 percent of Africans and Japanese, and 50 percent of certain tribes of Canadian Indians.

Recognizing the Symptoms

"Insidious" is perhaps the best way to describe the onset of AS. David is a typical patient. Now a young man in his early twenties, David came in for medical advice when he was a young teenager, suffering from pain in his back and legs. At the time the episodes of pain didn't make any sense. Whenever he pushed off to run, pain struck at the Achilles tendon in his heel like a sharp needle. Stiffness interfered with his life-style. David had *enthesopathy*; his ankle was tender where the tendon attached to the bone of the heel. This happens to AS sufferers wherever a tendon attaches to bone, and a sharp pain in the shoulders, buttocks, and backs of the knees is common.

Just as in rheumatoid arthritis, David developed pain in the lower back that was dull and aching at first. It was worse in the mornings and hurt enough that he had to get up early. The pain caused him to favor his back, and so he had trouble bending over to pick up things. He finally couldn't sleep at night because every time he stretched out on the bed, he couldn't stay on his back because of the pain. David only recently sought medical advice. Typical of AS sufferers, he kept thinking, *The pain is going to go away. It's just a strained muscle.*

By this time, my examination of David revealed that his back motion was severely restricted, and he was exquisitely tender over both sacroiliac joints where the spine joins the pelvis. He not only couldn't touch his toes while leaning over, but his lower back could have balanced a cup of coffee—it was so flat. Checking his heel cords with a pinch caused him to literally jump off the table with pain. His chest expansion was limited to the point that it was hard to tell whether he was breathing in or out. The lost motion of his ribs during breathing was due to the pain in the joints where the ribs meet the spine.

David was advised to go to the eye doctor for a checkup even though he had no symptoms or problems. Sure enough, he had an inflammation of the eye, called *iritis*, which is also common with AS. The front part of his eye had mildly inflamed as part of the rheumatic disease process.

David's experience is a classic example of AS. First, there is an insidious onset of vague lower back pain occurring over many months (more than three to meet the criteria for diagnosis). The pain is intermittent at first and then becomes more serious and constant. The initial pain is often very low in the back in the sacroiliac joints, which become extremely tender to pressure. Sometimes AS begins with pain and swelling of leg joints such as those in the hip or knee. Fatigue, weight loss, inactivity stiffness, and even a low-grade fever accompany the lower back pain. One major difference in the pain of AS as opposed to injury such as a ruptured disc is that, while disc pain is improved with rest, the pain of AS usually gets worse with rest and better with movement.

Additionally, the loss of motion in the lower spine is worsened by a flattening of the curve of the back when the body bends. The most important long-term worry with AS is that the joints connecting each vertebra will fuse together over time and the person will be hunched over. This is preventable with a strong and dedicated exercise program.

AS can also occur higher up in the neck and chest areas of the spine, but this occurs much less frequently. When the chest is involved the restriction of motion of the ribs interferes with proper breathing. The lungs are also affected, sometimes by scar tissue from the inflammation of AS. This, too, is preventable with proper exercise.

As indicated, other parts of the body can also be involved in AS. Iritis, or inflammation of the front part of the eye, is sudden in onset. Many times this is only found by an eye doctor since there are no symptoms. Iritis can be treated and is almost always mild. It doesn't last long or cause permanent injury.

The enthesopathy mentioned above is often a prominent feature of AS early on before the diagnosis is clear. The heel cord is the best example of an affected area, but it can happen anywhere in the body. The pain is often severe, but enthesopathy plus sacroiliac arthritis virtually makes the diagnosis of AS certain. Enthesopathy comes and goes, lasting a few weeks to a few months, and usually doesn't cause serious injury to the tendon or bone.

Finally, the heart valves of the aorta, the body's main blood vessel, which carries all of the blood from the heart, can be injured on rare occasion by AS, causing *aortic valve insufficiency*. Leakage of blood then occurs when the valve closes, making the heart work harder to pump the blood needed to maintain the body. If necessary, this can be corrected by surgery.

Investigating the Causes

As with rheumatoid arthritis, a genetic predisposition with a triggering event is the most likely cause of AS. In fact, the genetic causal evidence is stronger with AS than with RA, given that studies of people giving blood who were HLA-B27 positive revealed that 1 in 4 had symptoms of AS. Close relatives of HLA-B27-positive AS sufferers are at an increased risk for AS also. (See "Investigating the Causes" in chapter 1 for more information on genetic studies.)

There are some associated diseases that seem to be related to the HLA-B27-positive spectrum of disease. Reiter's syndrome victims are HLA-B27-positive people who experience arthritis, burning on urination, and red eyes. Many AS sufferers have episodes of burning on urination. Arthritis and inflammatory colitis, which causes chronic bloody diarrhea, occur in some people who are HLA-B27 positive.

The evidence is strong that HLA-B27 and AS are closely related. This intriguing relationship encouraged investigators recently to inject the HLA-B27 gene into a group of rats. The animals contracted chronic diarrhea first. The males then developed arthritis and genital problems. Injecting other HLA genes didn't cause arthritis or the other changes. So this model shows us that HLA-B27 is somehow related not only to AS but to Reiter's syndrome and chronic colitis.

Determining the Prognosis

It's difficult to get an accurate prognosis for AS because our knowledge of HLA antigenic genetic markers, and in particular HLA-B27, is now changing rapidly. The most important thing to know is that AS is usually active for about 10 years, but the damage it does to your spine, hips, or knees usually levels off after that. In studies of people with AS, the disease leveled off in almost all of them, but as many as 40 percent had restriction of joint motion of the spine. Twenty pecent will have arthritis of hips or knees, and occasionally other peripheral joints will remain painful. Those who developed AS as teenagers are more likely to have a hip replacement than those who developed AS after age 30. The older you were at onset, the less likely it is that you will have severe arthritis of the hips or knees. The good news for all ages is that there is joint replacement available to you even if the joint is bad.

AS iritis is usually mild, limited to a few weeks or months of inflammation and treatable with eye drops and occasionally steroids by mouth. Iritis rarely causes loss of visual acuity if the patient carefully follows the advice of an eye doctor for treatment and follow-up.

When AS does affect the heart and aorta, the aortic valve insufficiency previously mentioned can cause trouble, but surgical correction is possible. If the ribs become restricted in motion such that you don't move enough air in and out for proper health, this can lead to lung problems and scarring of the tissue. In many studies, the vast majority of AS sufferers had reduced ability to breathe properly and reduced pulmonary function. This too can be prevented by not allowing a loss of motion where the ribs join the spine.

A Course of Treatment

The outlook for AS actually is better than at first glance. Healthy living and exercise, helped by the NSAIDs, are the keys to success in your treatment. The earlier you begin a treatment program, the less trouble you will have. Don't wait until you've lost chest expansion or you can't straighten up any more. Like most things in life, it's easier to keep what you already have than recover what you've lost.

The first traditional advice to AS sufferers is to have a hard, firm bed and to sleep on your back. In fact, many people will swear by a half-inch plywood board placed under the mattress. However, as long as you practice an aggressive exercise program, you should use whatever mattress allows you to have the most restful sleep. This may mean that a firm waterbed may be better for a good night's sleep for you than a thick plywood board under your mattress if it keeps you awake.

Second, sitting upright in your chair with shoulders back and spine straight can help to keep you from feeling like the hunch-back of Notre Dame. If your work is sedentary, be sure that your chair doesn't place a strain on you; use a special chair if you want to protect your back. Move around frequently during the day; don't let yourself get too stiff.

There are no special foods that help AS, but a sensible diet that balances your intake of calories with your output of calories is essential. Above all, keep your weight down, and if you're over-weight, get rid of it. Remember that when you run or jump, every pound of weight translates into 4 to 8 pounds of pressure on the joints.

Here is an example of a success story. Tom was HLA–B27 positive and had arthritis of the spine with onset of AS as an adolescent. I counseled him over a period of years about exercising and choosing a career that would not involve lifting heavy objects. Tom established a daily routine of doing situps and swimming. To improve his lung capacity he took up the trumpet and clarinet. During high school he and some of his friends organized a country western band. When I last saw Tom, he was making a living with a band in the Austin area and had a place on the Guadelupe

River, where he did his situps every morning and then swam. His back motion was fine, and so was he.

Thinking ahead, planning ahead, and using the tools at your disposal are essential not only to your well-being but to your survival. Consider first what kind of exercise you need for your back and legs. Ideally, you should maintain and improve normal motion in your back. Situps and stretching exercises for the back on a Roman chair are examples of strengthening and stretching exercises using equipment in a health club situation. Deep-breathing exercise twice daily can also include blowing up balloons to maintain motion in the ribs.

The best exercise eliminates pressure on the joints while building strength and endurance in the muscles and stretching the ligaments around the joints. Water exercise can be invaluable. Walking around the pool in deep water in your AquaJogger is a good way to get started. The first day aquajog only a few minutes and increase the time daily. This is a sensible way to increase strength and endurance for the rest of the day. We'll discuss more on this topic in chapter 13.

If exercise in the water is not an option, a daily exercise program outlined by an exercise trainer in a health club is essential. If you are fortunate and have an interested physical therapist who can follow your progress, do so.

Concerning medications, NSAIDs are essential to relieving pain. You cannot follow a proper exercise program in the presence of serious pain. These medicines also reduce the inflammation in the joints of the back and the legs. Many arthritis doctors believe that some NSAIDs, including indomethacin, work better than others in relieving the pain of AS. The toxic side effects are serious; any drug must be given under close medical supervision. Other NSAIDs such as Naprosyn are often tried first before indomethacin is given. Chapter 10 contains more details on medications.

If necessary, joint replacement of the hip or knee has made life enormously more productive for literally thousands of sufferers for many years now. We'll explore this option in greater detail in chapter 18.

While not strictly a necessary part of treatment, genetic counseling can be useful for your family. Some researchers postulate that AS skips a generation, but there is no confirming information on this observation. You may wish, however, to talk about the chances of your children having AS later in life. Three of 10 close relatives of people with AS will develop AS. You and your significant other need to work through your feelings on this important matter if you are contemplating children.

Insurance, both health and life, will be a major concern for you unless there is an overhaul in the health care system in our country. Don't change jobs or insurance carriers until you have assurance in writing that coverage will be provided for your AS.

Most people don't realize the importance of ordinary health and living habits. If you're a smoker, stop right now. Smoking will destroy your lungs, and with AS possibly restricting your breathing, you need all the help you can get. Smoking also injures your heart and blood vessels.

Finally, there are two voluntary organizations that can keep you up to date on AS: the Arthritis Foundation and the Ankylosing Spondylitis Association. The addresses are given in Appendix 1. Join both to get the best continuing information.

5

Osteoporosis

Osteoporosis means "porous bone." Its medical significance is that the bone has lost both calcium for strength and matrix for support. The bone becomes too fragile to withstand ordinary stresses, and a fracture typically results. Osteoporosis is a major cause of serious disability in older people, with one in three women and one in five men living to age 85 fracturing a hip due to osteoporosis. Another term interchangeably used is *osteopenia*.

Bone has several reasons for existence in our bodies. It provides a frame for support, allows us to move around in our environment, protects us from being banged around, and is a storing place for many of the basic chemicals essential for the normal functioning of the body. It's composed of many minerals, the most important being calcium for strength, and 70 percent of it is composed of a soft, supporting material called collagen. Bone is not simply a girder of calcium that forms the skeleton like the supports of a building; it is a dynamic organ like the heart or kidneys, with thousands of chemical reactions going on continuously. Bone is changing and remodeling every minute of the day. As children, our bones grow from growth plates of cartilage at the ends of bones. Bone turnover rates in growing children can be 20 percent yearly. In adults the turnover rate is still 3 to 5 percent yearly. After we reach adulthood, remodeling continues, whether it is healing that occurs after a fracture, or an ever-changing equilibrium of calcium being added and taken away to maintain strength.

There are many checks and balances in our skeletal system. Hormones such as parathyroid and vitamins such as vitamin D control the level of calcium in bone. Cortisone from the adrenal glands and medicines containing cortisone drugs cause loss of calcium from bones. Growth hormone increases the collagen supporting tissue of bone. The sex hormones exert a large force; at menopause the loss of estrogen causes a rapid loss of bone. What this adds up to is that the constant remodeling of bone is the sum of the interaction of hormones and mechanical stresses of life on the basic growth centers of bones. It is a constant, dynamic equilibrium.

What Is Osteoporosis?

Osteoporosis is the excessive loss of calcium and matrix of bone. It is usually elusive and discovered only because a fracture occurs after minimal trauma, and an X ray shows a washed-out image of the bone. It is sometimes noticed because the person shows reduced height or a humping of the back, or suffers from low back pain.

Dr. Bevra Hahn and her husband, Dr. Theodore Han, medical researchers of osteoporosis for many years, point out that bone loss begins as early as 20 years old and is over three times greater in women than in men. Osteoporosis is a serious problem to be reckoned with among older folks. About 25 million people in our country are afflicted, most of whom are women. In fact, it affects half of all women over the age of 45 years, and 90 percent of women over 75 years. The American Academy of Orthopedic Surgeons estimates that osteoporosis causes over one million fractures yearly, and that one-third of women and one-fifth of men living to age 85 will have a fracture of the hip due to osteoporosis.

One reason that men have less osteoporosis than women is that men have more total bone mass. Studies show that after age 40 all of us lose bone at one-half percent yearly; in women, however, the loss doubles after the onset of menopause. Adding to the problem for women is that the calcium balance of what comes in and what goes out becomes negative at a rate two times higher than before menopause.

Causes

As we get older, less bone is made, and more bone is lost. Our genetic heritage is one factor, although there can also be problems with absorbing food properly, caused by such factors as inadequate intake of vitamins and calcium. Hormone excess such as too much parathyroid or thyroid hormone can cause loss of calcium. Too much steroid medicine also causes loss of calcium from the bone.

As mentioned above, menopause—in particular, premature menopause before age 45—causes a sharp reduction in estrogen hormones, which results in an accelerated loss of bone. There are associated factors that need attention if present to reduce osteoporosis: too little physical activity, low intake of vitamin D, inadequate exposure to sunlight, use of tobacco, and excessive alcohol use.

Prognosis

Until recently, the outlook for people with osteoporosis was gloomy. It seemed like a fact of life, and the sheer number of sufferers—25 million Americans—was a testimony to its seeming inevitability. With an estimated 1.3 million fractures yearly (half of women over the age of 50 have an osteoporosis-related fracture), osteoporosis is a major health issue. Indeed, as many as 35,000 older people who sustain fractures of the spine, hips, or arms due to osteoporosis die yearly of complications.

Today, however, much more is known about preventing osteoporosis, and most people can limit its devasting effects. Studies from the Mayo Clinic especially offer hope.

A Course of Treatment

Prevention is the main treatment, of which exercise, healthy living—including proper amounts of calcium and vitamin D in the diet—and estrogen treatment for women are the keys to success. Let's look at each of these treatments.

Exercise. We now know that muscle mass and bone formation increase with exercise, even in older people. It especially helps to exercise against gravity, such as walking a mile or more daily or at least several times weekly. Arranging and following a program in a health club outlined by an exercise trainer will help you achieve the most benefit to your body within your limitations. You can also improve your endurance and strength by exercising in the water with such things as the AquaJogger, which offers you buoyancy, versatility, and freedom to exercise in the uniquely resistant and impact-free environment of water. Several companies are now making weights that attach to ankles or wrists for use in water. See chapter 13 for details about exercise.

Healthy living. A proper diet that contains adequate vitamin D (about 400 international units daily) and calcium (about 1,000 miligrams daily, 1,500 miligrams daily for postmenopausal women) is essential. Vitamin D, of course, is plentiful from the sun, so walking outdoors probably takes care of this, but an older person might take a daily multivitamin that includes trace elements of minerals. Calcium can be obtained from food, with milk and cheese high on the list, but many other foods, such as broccoli, and fish, such as salmon and sardines, provide as much as a fifth of daily requirements in usual portions. (See Figure 2 for different foods rich in calcium.) If you're not able to eat these calcium-containing foods, calcium tablets may be substituted. They come in many kinds of preparations and are sold across the counter with no prescription needed. Look on the label to see how much is in the tablet and decide how much to take based on how much calcium-rich food you eat. (The price of the tablets varies considerably in different preparations.) One problem with oral calcium is that the preparations can make you a little nauseous or queasy. So only buy a small bottle and try out *one* tablet first to see if it agrees with your body. Check with your doctor to see which brand he or she prefers, if any.

Estrogen treatment. Estrogens are useful not only to prevent osteoporosis but also to treat it. As mentioned earlier, bone loss in women after menopause doubles, so taking estrogen at menopause makes sense. In a recent study by the Mayo Clinic of postmenopausal women, estrogen was administered to about 40 women using a skin-patch system, while about 35 like women received no estrogen. The women receiving estrogen increased calcium in their bones by 7 percent, but more important, they had one-half the number of fractures.

The importance of this study is that for the first time, there is good evidence that estrogens not only help prevent osteoporosis from happening, but can be used to reduce the number of fractures caused by brittle, osteoporotic bone. However, like most

Figure 2
Foods Rich in Calcium
National Dairy Council

	250+ mg	150–249 mg	70–149 mg
MILK GROUP: foods rich in calcium, riboflavin, protein	**Milks** Buttermilk 285 mg Chocolate 280 mg Malted 347 Whole 291 mg 1% lowfat 300 mg 2% lowfat 297 mg Skim 302 mg **Cheeses** Ricotta, part skim 337 mg Swiss 302 mg Milkshakes Chocolate 396 mg Vanilla 457 mg **Yogurts. Lowfat** Flavored 389 mg Fruit 345 mg Plain 415 mg	**Cheeses** American, pasteurized 174 mg Blue 150 mg Caraway 191 mg Cheddar 204 mg Cheese food American, pasteurized process 163 mg Swiss, pasteurized process 205 mg Colby 194 mg Edam 207 mg Monterey 212 mg Mozzarella, part skim, low moisture 203 mg Muenster 203 mg	**Cheese** Cottage, 2% lowfat 78 mg **Frozen desserts** Ice cream 88 mg Ice milk, hardened 88 mg Ice milk, soft serve 137 mg Pudding, chocolate 146 mg Beans, dried, cooked 90 mg Shrimp, canned 98 mg Tofu 108 mg
MEAT GROUP: foods rich in protein, niacin, iron, thiamin	Sardines, with bones 371 mg	Salmon, with bones 167 mg	
GRAIN GROUP: foods rich in carbohydrate, thiamin, iron, niacin		Waffle 179 mg	Pancakes 72 mg

★ Figures are based on what are generally accepted to be usual portions.

good things in life, there's a down side here. Estrogens are associated with a slightly increased incidence of cancer of the breast and uterus, but most people feel that the trade-off is worth it. You and your doctor will have to decide.

Another drug used to treat osteoporosis is calcitonin. The evidence for its use is not as clear as estrogen or calcium, so ask your doctor about this medicine.

In the long run, your best bet is to prevent osteoporosis to the best of your ability, especially if there is a genetic trait in your family. Following these three suggestions can improve your quality of life.

6

Other Rheumatic Diseases

Rheumatic diseases are not limited to arthritis. Some involve other tissues and organs of the body but can cause arthritis to a lesser degree. The main problems in the treatment of these diseases are not related to inflammation of the joints and loss of motion and strength due to arthritis, but to other issues that the disease brings to light.

This chapter reviews two of these relatively rare rheumatic diseases: *systemic lupus erythematosus* and *gout*. There are also *polymyositis/dermatomyositis,* which is a chronic inflammatory of the muscles primarily with little if any arthritis, and *scleroderma,* which is a rare rheumatic condition characterized by hardness of the skin and supporting structures with systemic involvement of many organs.

These two diseases are rare, and we unfortunately lack the space to detail them.

What Is
Systemic Lupus Erythematosus?

Like rheumatoid arthritis, systemic lupus erythematosus (SLE) is a chronic inflammatory disease of the joints. It is also a disease that involves virtually every other organ of the body, including the skin, kidneys, heart, nerves, brain, and blood. It seems to originate in the immune system of the body, which somehow turns on itself and produces antibodies that participate in injuring or destroying a wide variety of tissues. There are autoantibodies called antinuclear antibodies that for reasons unknown are formed against normal nuclear materials of the body's own cells. They occur in the vast majority of people with SLE as well as in those with other autoimmune diseases. The presence of these antibodies and other characteristics of lupus separates SLE from other rheumatic diseases.

Fortunately, the disease is rare, with only about 100,000 people in our country afflicted. SLE strikes mainly young women under 30, and about 90 percent of all cases are women. There are also ethnic differences, with African-Americans, Hispanics, and Orientals affected three to five times more than white groups.

Recognizing the Symptoms

The usual victim of lupus is a young woman who experiences over a period of months increasing fatigue, weight loss, a low-grade fever, and pain in the joints with little or no swelling. Soon she also experiences painful swelling of a few joints, leading physicians astray, since many other conditions also share these symptoms. In about half the people with SLE, a peculiar butterfly rash occurs on the face that in the old days was likened to a wolf face, hence the name *lupus*. The antinuclear antibody blood test is indicated at this point and is highly positive.

What happens next to this individual is so variable that doctors cannot draw a typical road map of disease progression. SLE mimics almost every disease we know, and any or all of the following can happen: Inflammation of the kidney causes blood in the urine with serious resulting damage to the kidney, called glomerulonephritis. In addition to the butterfly rash, other changes in the skin occur such as loss of hair (alopecia) and photosensitivity to the rays of the sun, causing serious rashes.

Fluid can also collect around the heart, lungs, or intestines, causing pressure and sometimes misleading the doctor into thinking cancer is the cause. The liver and spleen are at times enlarged. SLE attacks the red blood cells, resulting in anemia, and a low white-blood-cell count and low platelet count are also common. The brain can be involved, and seizures can occur.

Lupus also causes arthritis, although the pain is usually not as severe as with RA. (Destructive arthritis is rare.) Pain in the muscles is also common but is not serious. Inflammation of the blood vessels can cause spasms of the tiny blood vessels of the fingers, for example, producing whiteness and coldness of the skin with pain, called Raynaud's phenomenon. This occurs particularly when the hands are exposed to cold, and the inflammation can be severe enough that the blood supply to a finger is shut off, causing serious injury.

However, the patterns of the course of SLE are quite variable. All of the above problems occur in up to half of sufferers of SLE at some point in their illness.

Investigating the Causes

Like all rheumatic diseases, the cause or causes of lupus are unknown today. Abnormalities of the immune system undoubtedly are a factor, but whether these changes are a primary cause or simply a reaction of the body to injury is unclear. There does appear to be a genetic predisposition to lupus, but it is not as strong as the genetic factor behind RA. Identical twins are known to have SLE, but there are other identical twins where only one had the disease. The association of SLE in young women of childbearing age is clear, so one might guess that hormonal influences are a factor too. Many drugs can induce SLE; most of them are commonly used in other diseases. SLE disappears when the offending drug is stopped. In animal experimental models, certain foods have had an effect on SLE. Alfalfa sprouts have produced a disease very much like SLE in monkeys. Diets that are high in oils from certain cold-water fish containing eicosanoic acid, when fed to autoimmune mice, appear to help the nephritis produced by their autoimmune disease. This has led to an interest in using cold-water fish oils to treat lupus.

Determining the Prognosis

Before the advent of corticosteroids, the mortality rate was high for lupus, with the majority of people with serious kidney disease dying and those without renal disease surviving in only 50 percent of cases. With the widespread use of steroid treatments for SLE, the survival rate for people without serious renal problems is now more than 90 percent, and for people with serious nephritis, it is about 70 percent. The arthritis effect is seldom a serious problem, other than self-limited pain, and destructive arthritis is unusual. The other organs such as the heart and brain can incur serious illness, but the kidney is usually the prime organ to be severely affected.

A Course of Treatment for SLE

The main treatment for lupus is steroid medicine. Unfortunately, because the doses are high, serious side effects are frequent. The cytotoxic drugs—azathioprine, cyclophosphamide, and methotrexate—are given to the most seriously ill people with SLE.

NSAIDs are used for sufferers who have a mild disease to treat pain and provide an anti-inflammatory effect on the joints. Hydroxychloroquine is used for the skin rash and arthritis of SLE, but people are advised to protect themselves from the sun to reduce photosensitivity.

What Is Gout?

Gout is an acute and chronic inflammatory arthritis mainly occurring in 30- to 60-year-old men. Fewer than 1 in 10 are women. Estimates vary, but over 500,000 people have gout. We know that gout is caused by sodium monourate crystals that collect in the joint fluid, which can cause terrible pain and swelling of joints; the big toe is often severely afflicted. One indication of gout is that too much uric acid is produced by the body or too little is excreted by the kidney; either condition results in too much uric acid in the body, including the joints. There is also a related disease, *pseudogout,* which is in the same disease family but linked to another chemical in the body called calcium pyrophosphate dihydrate (CPPD).

Many associated events can trigger an acute episode, including high blood pressure, excessive drinking, being overweight, and even love of foods rich in purines (proteins that are important sources of uric acid) such as glandular meats (sweetbreads). Stress or an associated illness can also trigger an attack.

One of the primary symptoms of gout is lumps under the skin, called *tophi*, around the elbows, heels, or ears. These are caused by urate crystals which fill the lumps. The diagnosis of gout is made by looking at the crystals under a microscope that are taken either from joint fluid or from a *tophus*.

The treatment of gout is a great success story. By controlling the level of uric acid with medicines, and using NSAIDs to reduce the pain of an acute attack, doctors have been able to achieve a high success rate. Colchicine is used as a primary way to reduce attacks and is taken propylactically by mouth. Another great advance was the discovery of ways to control the level of uric acid in the blood, thereby reducing gout attacks. If a gout sufferer is an overproducer of uric acid, doctors use a medicine called allopurinol (Zyloprim) that blocks the production of uric acid. If too little uric acid is being excreted by the kidney, medicines are given that increase excretion in the urine, such as probenecid (Benemid) and sulfinpyrazone (Anturane).

The outlook for gout sufferers is excellent if they stick to a serious regimen of weight control, eat sensibly, refrain from excessive alcohol, and take the medicines as prescribed by the doctor.

7

Juvenile Rheumatoid Arthritis

Contrary to common belief, arthritis does occur in children and teenagers. In fact, I have spent my professional life taking care of young people with arthritis. Juvenile rheumatoid arthritis (JRA) is one of at least a hundred kinds of chronic arthritis that can afflict children, and it is the most common one. Recent national health care statistics reveal that up to 200,000 children have arthritis of some kind and at least half of that number have JRA. This means that arthritis in the young is twice as common as diabetes. Our discussion here will focus on the basic facts. For further information, consult our previous book, *Parenting a Child with Arthritis* (Lowell House, 1992).

What Is
Juvenile Rheumatoid Arthritis?

JRA is chronic arthritis of childhood with swelling, pain, and tenderness of at least one joint and lasting longer than six weeks with no other cause apparent to the doctor.

Let's refer back to chapter 1 (rheumatoid arthritis) and apply the important information presented there to JRA. Juvenile rheumatoid arthritis is an active, inflammatory, peripheral, symmetrical arthritis afflicting three girls for every boy. *Active* means that JRA is an ongoing process lasting for years. *Inflammatory* indicates swelling, redness, tenderness, and pain in the joints. *Peripheral* tells us that JRA involves mainly the joints of the arms and legs, in particular the fingers and wrists. *Symmetrical* provides a key to tell the disease apart from a lot of other kinds of arthritis. JRA usually involves the same joints on both sides of the body—the knees, wrists, or joints of the fingers, for example. Add to that, *stiffness* of the joints after inactivity and the requirement that arthritis last six weeks or longer in the same joints, and we have the official American College of Rheumatology definition for *juvenile rheumatoid arthritis.*

The onset of JRA—that is, what happens in the beginning months of disease—is a clue to which of the three types of JRA a child may develop: *pauciarticular* JRA (four or fewer joints with arthritis), *polyarticular* JRA (five joints or more with arthritis), or *systemic* JRA (spiking fever and rheumatoid rash). There is also a small group of JRA boys who have pauci JRA, usually with arthritis in the joints of the legs, who often have heel pain and inflammation of the heel tendons (tenosynovitis). These boys are also HLA-B27 positive (see chapter 4). Let's examine these three types of JRA.

Pauciarticular. Pauciarticular JRA is the mildest form, and about 45 percent of JRA children have pauciarticular JRA. Children with this type have very few joints swollen, usually in the legs. Pauciarticular JRA kids are usually girls younger than 10 years of age.

Mary, a five-year-old kindergarten student, experienced pain and discomfort off and on in her knee for several weeks. One day her mother noticed that the knee was swollen a bit and that Mary could no longer straighten her leg. After a week or two, she noticed that one or two other joints had also become swollen. In the mornings Mary's leg was stiff for about an hour after she got up. She also ran a low-grade fever on many days. When Mary and her mother visited the eye doctor he found mild iritis, and prompt treatment controlled it. Only 5 to 10 percent of children with JRA develop iritis; most of them are in the pauciarticular group, and almost all are girls.

Polyarticular. About 1 child in 4 has polyarticular JRA, or arthritis in five joints or more within six months of onset. These children have fever and swelling in many joints. The vast majority are girls who are older than the children with pauciarticular or systemic onset. Many of the polyarticular JRA children have a positive rheumatoid factor (RF) in their blood, indicating arthritis. Again, RF is a special antibody related to the gamma globulin proteins of the blood that is positive in almost all adults with RA.

Children with polyarticular JRA, many of whom test RF positive, often have enlarged lymph nodes (under the arms, for example) and develop lumps under the skin called *subcutaneous nodules*. These movable lumps are not painful, are usually located around the elbows, wrists, forearms, shins, ankles, or feet, and are attached to the covering of the bones or other deep tissue. They are harmless, lasting usually a few months and then disappearing; although in my experience, patients with these nodules have more trouble with their arthritis later. The liver may also be slightly enlarged, though it does not cause problems. Polyarticular JRA is potentially most destructive to the joints and calls for an active and aggressive treatment with medicines and physical therapy.

Systemic. About 30 percent of children with JRA have the systemic form of the disease, and unlike pauci or poly JRA, boys are affected in the same numbers as girls.

"Explosive" is the best way to describe the beginning of systemic JRA. A typical story is that of six-year old Cindy, who awoke one night with a 105 degree fever. Horrified, her mother saw a splotchy, salmon-pink rash on Cindy's body and face that disappeared and reappeared. Every joint in her body was painful and swollen. For Cindy and many children like her, hospitalization is required at this early stage. Many tests are done in search of the cause, though eventually the spiking fever and intermittent rash lead to a diagnosis of JRA.

Several organs in the body can be affected by systemic JRA. The sac around the heart may fill with fluid; and the liver, spleen, and lymph nodes may enlarge. Even the kidneys do not escape unscathed, and blood cells are found in the urine. Serious anemia often shows up and causes fatigue. White blood cells are markedly increased in the blood count, causing further concern about infection.

The intermittent or spiking fever of systemic JRA is and can be greater than 103 degrees, lasting a few hours in the evening before returning to normal. One or two episodes occur each day. The spiking fever can resemble that which occurs in a serious infection. For this reason, exhaustive tests are needed to rule out infection if the characteristic rash is absent.

The rash that usually accompanies the JRA fever is one of the strangest things you'll ever see. Salmon-pink and smooth, with clearly defined, irregular borders, it varies in size from a small button to several inches in diameter with a pale center. Located anywhere on the body but most often on the trunk and face, it moves around and comes and goes in minutes. Occasionally the rash itches, or it may be raised. It is considered a vascular rash and in itself is not injurious to the body.

A less obvious problem is fluid around the heart or, more accurately, inside the sac around the heart. No symptoms or discomfort is present, and only through an ultrasound test, the echocardiogram, can the fluid be detected. Unless your child has symptoms such as shortness of breath or chest pain, or your doctor hears a rubbing sound over the heart through the stethoscope, in general you need not worry. Even if pericarditis occurs, it is treatable and rarely life-threatening, and usually only lasts a few weeks or months.

Investigating the Causes

There are many theories about the causes of JRA, but no answers. Some genetic predisposition is involved. The immune and defense systems of the body somehow are not working properly, though infection as a triggering mechanism can't be dismissed. But it is important to remember that if you are a parent of a child with JRA, *you did not cause it!*

Increasing knowledge of genes and gene markers points to the probability that inherited genes predispose some people to certain types of JRA. In 30 years of practice, I saw many families with three and even four generations of rheumatic disease. Occurrence in a family, however, does not prove that it's inherited. The family could have been exposed to something in the environment that is the true cause.

Several studies also report high frequencies of severe stress at onset of JRA. This may be due to a divorce or separation of the child's parents, a death of a family member, or adoption. Time after time, mothers told me about the onset of JRA in their children following a recent divorce or separation. "It's almost like God was getting even," or "It came on too fast after the separation to be an accident," they said.

Another striking association with the onset of JRA is severe injury. While no one thinks that trauma causes the JRA, injury can trigger a disease flare-up. A teenage boy who was a patient in our center developed arthritis after falling off a truck as it swung around a corner. He did not break any bones but developed severe arthritis in virtually all joints at the moment of impact. His illness continued for several years.

Immunizations such as those for rubella or DTP (diptheria-tetanus-pertussis) produce an antibody response and can precipitate the onset of a chronic arthritis that is indistinguishable from JRA. Indeed, many experts believe that infections such as flu, infectious mono, or Lyme disease cause a reactive arthritis, meaning that the body develops arthritis as a reaction to the illness, much in the way serum sickness is a response to chemicals such as penicillin. Children who develop this kind of arthritis usually have a short duration of joint swelling in terms of a few weeks.

Note, however, that there is no such thing as a JRA personality. For many years noted psychologists and rheumatologists wrote and worried about a "rheumatoid personality" predisposing children to JRA. The personality characteristics described included depression, hostility, and difficulty in expressing anger. Controlled studies done in Houston comparing asthmatic children with JRA children revealed no "rheumatoid" personality; these personality traits are shared by all children already afflicted with a painful, chronic illness.

Determining the Prognosis

Most pauci JRA children continue their courses of disease with only one or two joints swollen, and after one or two years have no further trouble. These children are the lucky ones. There are, however, a few children who have a long-lasting disease with many joints involved, and thus require the most attention, a good exercise program, and the proper medication. Poly JRA kids are more likely to have some functional loss of motion of the joints. They will need to work diligently to minimize this through exercise, diet, and good health. If proper care is taken, these children can grow up, get a job, marry, and live independently. In the case of systemic JRA, if the child is lucky to have only one or two inflamed joints, the course of the disease will be like pauci JRA with little risk of iritis. The terrible fever and annoying rash do go away, and the heart almost never becomes a permanent problem even if pericarditis develops. If many joints are involved, it will be necessary to work doubly hard because of a greater risk of damage to the bone and cartilage of the joints and loss of normal use. For reasons that are not clear, JRA children in Europe, including Eastern Europe, have what is called amyloidosis which can cause death due to kidney failure in about 1 in 20 children. It is very rare in North America, and in over 30 years of practice, I did not see a single American JRA with amyloidosis. Death in JRA children in the United States is about 1 percent and is usually due to heart disease, infection, or an adverse reaction from a medicine.

A Course of Treatment

The best treatment for JRA is family-centered, community-based, and coordinated care. Family-centered care means that the family makes a joint effort to combat the disease. Since the family is directly affected by this serious, chronic illness, they must pull together to win the battle against JRA's effects. The family, including the JRA child, does what is necessary to help but does not let JRA take over and rule. In community-based care, community services to help children with JRA, such as physical therapy and special school services, must be not only in place but available at an affordable cost. Coordinated care means that a unified group works with the family to intelligently plan and coordinate appropriate health services and medicines needed at the appropriate times. This team should include a pediatric rheumatologist, nurse, social worker, nutritionist, and physical and occupational therapists. It should also include a counselor to help the child through school. Such a team can make the difference between success and failure.

Physical exercise to maintain strength and size of muscles and to improve endurance is essential for growing children. Exercise helps to prevent loss of joint motion. Splints can be used to protect joints such as the wrist from drifting to one side or to increase joint motion by gradually straightening joints such as the knee. For JRA children with serious problems in the hips, joint replacement by an orthopedist has been a godsend.

The same rules for taking NSAIDs in general apply to children with JRA as they do to adults with RA. Second-line drugs such as cortisone, gold, and methotrexate are used in much the same way in children as they are in adults, with the exception that since children are still growing, drugs such as cortisone derivatives can cause problems with growth. For this reason, drug therapy must be tailored to each child's specific needs.

With coordinated care and continuous support, children with JRA have the best chance for living a well-adjusted to life and entering the mainstream of adulthood with hope and confidence.

Part Two

BUILDING

A

TEAM

P art 1 of this book was devoted to helping you understand the many illnesses that fall under the category of rheumatic diseases. In Part 2 we will look at how you can take charge of your arthritis and make your life work. You are who you are; you may also be a mother, a father, an office manager, or the president of a successful company. You may also happen to have arthritis. Please don't ever think of or describe yourself as "arthritic." You are a *person* who happens to have arthritis, and how you deal with that arthritis will reveal a lot about what kind of person you are.

We would like to tell you about one of our heroes who has arthritis. When we organized the first annual meeting of the American Juvenile Arthritis Organization in Keystone, Colorado, about 10 years ago, we had no idea what the response would be. But we felt very strongly that there was a need for families of children with arthritis and the health professionals who treat them to get together and share their common experiences.

A young man living in Australia read about the conference and was determined to attend. He contacted Qantas Airlines and with his enthusiasm convinced them to fly him and his mother, free of charge, to the meeting—by way of Disneyland, of course. Benjamin was 14 years old and in a wheelchair. Several doctors had told him that the damage to his joints from his arthritis was so severe that he would not be able to walk until he matured and joint replacements could be performed. Thus he resigned himself to life in a wheelchair. When Ben arrived at the meeting, he was in for a pleasant surprise. For the first time, he met many other children with arthritis. There were crutches, braces, splints, electrical carts, and wheelchairs everywhere. Ben and his newfound friends enjoyed a good deal of commiserating with one another and joking about the stupid things people said to them ("*Children* don't get arthritis!"). Well, Ben had a terrific time and went home with a renewed vitality.

The next year he came to the organization's second annual meeting in St. Louis, Missouri. Ben was *walking!* Astounded, Kathy asked his mother if it was because of the drugs, and she smiled and shook her head. "It was Ben! Only Ben!" she said proudly. She told me that after the first meeting Ben realized that other children with arthritis were walking, so why wasn't he? He had found a new determination. He began swimming, physical therapy, and weight training. He told his mother that if he dropped something, she should leave it there—if he wanted it badly enough he would find a way to get it!

At the second meeting, Ben pushed *other* children in their wheelchairs, telling them not to give up, not to believe everything they are told, not to rely on a wheelchair all the time. Remember the story we told earlier about the bumblebee who flew even though it didn't know that it wasn't supposed to fly? Ben was the best example of that anecdote come to life. This 14-year-old decided to listen to his own heart, and he was able to accomplish an incredible feat. Although the doctors' X rays showed severe damage to his joints, and it seemed that it would be impossible for someone with that kind of damage to walk, those X rays could not look into Ben's soul, the spirit of this child. I have faith that Ben will probably be the prime minister of Australia someday!

Don't let other people set limits on your capabilities. Don't set limits on your own abilities. If you don't *try* you will never know if you *can!*

Part 2 of this book is about how you can become a bumblebee. You'll learn about setting your own goals and finding ways to achieve them. Physicians, drugs, therapists, and therapies of all sorts are simply means to an end—that end being a happy, productive life. I don't know a single person who does not have some cross to bear in this lifetime. Some are heavier than others, but we each have our own. You have been given a special challenge, so don't be shy about asking for help. In the final analysis, it is *your* challenge. Good luck!

8

The First Member of Your Team Is You!

OK, so you have arthritis. Just what are you going to do about it? You didn't ask for it, you certainly don't want it, but it doesn't seem to want to go away. Clearly, one way to take control is to get help from a doctor. There are many wonderful health professionals out there who have spent their lives helping people with arthritis. You need to get a diagnosis, learn about what type of arthritis you have, and find out what the probable outcome will be. That evaluation will be made by the physician you choose. He or she may be a rheumatologist, an internist, or a family practitioner. This person should have access to a variety of other health professionals to help you work toward your goal of a normal life. You need to have coordinated, comprehensive, continuous care. Obviously, it is extremely important that all of these people be able to communicate with one another as well as with you.

The idea of having a team of health professionals is a fairly recent innovation in medicine. With chronic diseases it is virtually impossible for one person to meet the tremendous variety of needs of each patient. I had a dear friend in Houston, Helga, who had rheumatoid arthritis. When she was first diagnosed I had been helping my 14-year-old daughter, Elizabeth, fight her battle with arthritis for several years. Helga had seen the amount of physical therapy Elizabeth received morning and night, including the hot paraffin bath in which I warmed my daughter's hands and feet to alleviate her pain. Helga knew that Elizabeth tried to swim in a heated pool whenever possible. She was aware that there were *many* things going on around our house to keep Elizabeth active and involved in school.

By contrast, the only thing Helga's physician did was prescribe medication. Helga did not understand why she was so fatigued, why she was so cold much of the time, why she had difficulty getting out of bed some mornings. She would call me for information because she didn't want to "bother" her doctor by asking him such "minor" questions. Now I would ask you, is not being able to get out of bed a "minor" problem? This doctor definitely needed at the very least a good nurse and a physical therapist to help Helga understand just what was happening to her body and how to handle the problems she was facing. That is the role of a health team: to educate, to coordinate, to help you live a normal life. But remember, this is a collaborative effort with *you* in the lead.

You are going to have to do a great deal of soul searching, which is not a bad thing to do. Many people rush headlong through life with no real objectives and find at the end of their lives that they have wasted much of their talent. You will now be forced to really look at your life and decide just what is important and what can be deleted. A diagnosis of arthritis is not the end of your life. There are many things you can do to keep control of your daily activities. It will take more self-discipline than you may be used to. Where exercise might have once been an overlooked drudgery, it now becomes an imperative aspect of life. Weight control is important in managing certain pain and in generally diminishing stress to your joints, so good nutrition will also become a newfound phrase. Relaxation techniques take on a whole new meaning in helping to ease the pain of arthritis.

You as Team Leader

Your goal, despite having arthritis, is to live a normal, fulfilling life. Each of us has our own concept of exactly what that goal might be. In order to reach your goal, you will need to assemble a team to assist you in your effort. Available resources will depend to a great extent on where you live. In large cities medical help will be more readily available. Many rheumatologists in large medical centers work as part of a team of health professionals. In smaller communities health professionals such as physical therapists, nutritionists, and psychologists, may not be an immediate part of the physician's team, but your doctor or nurse will probably know of people to whom they can refer you. The nurse in a rural area may perform other duties, including counseling or teaching range-of-motion exercises. Also, the size of smaller towns may allow easier accessibility to professional help.

Again, the most important member of your team is *you*. Say we create a list of all the possible ways of coping with arthritis: going to a physician, taking medication, exercising, eating properly, resting, seeking help for any emotional problems, finding someone to help you with an exercise program, having surgical replacements, and so forth. When you look at the list, you will realize that the only one who can implement these things, the only one who can begin the process of healing, is *you!* You have to make that first appointment. *You* have to do the exercises, take the medicine, listen to your body, and act accordingly. The good news is that you are not alone. There are a multitude of people out there to help you. But *you* have to ask for help.

What Are Friends for Anyway?

The next important members of your team are your family and friends. The very fact that they care about you means they will also be impacted by your arthritis. Because arthritis is usually a long-term battle, you will need a lot of support from those around you. Even the strongest people will have bad days, days in which they will need a friendly shoulder to lean on. When it seems impossible to get out of bed because your joints feel like hardened cement, you will need a friend to gently give you a shove toward that hot bath or shower. You will need them to help on those dark days, and to celebrate on those days of victory!

Andrea, a woman approaching 40, tells me that when she was diagnosed with rheumatoid arthritis at the age of 18, she totally denied that she had a problem. She just muddled through the best way she could, with little help. Today she has serious impairment, probably in part from the years of neglect. She has a loving, caring family, and she admits that if she had gathered support from them in those early years of the disease, she would probably not be as impaired as she is today. We will never know. But if you are newly diagnosed, don't repeat Andrea's mistake. Don't look back in 20 years and wish you had done things differently. The resources are there. Use them for your benefit!

Let your family and friends know that you are afraid. Tell them that you don't want to be dependent on others. Tell them your anxiety about the possible side effects of the medications you must take. If you share your deepest thoughts with those who care, they can help you work toward solutions. Family members can help with the day-to-day necessary things—physical therapy, medications, encouragement, and just being there.

It is really horrible to love someone and see them in pain. Parents who have had to watch their children scream in pain with arthritis have said that they wish they had the arthritis instead. I was one of them. Your family members will understand your suffering as no one else will. And pain is difficult for all of us to live with. It produces all sorts of negative feelings and destructive fears.

Dealing with Fear

You must overcome your fears in order to be an effective team leader. A good place to start is to first acknowledge their existence. We'll focus on some of the more prevalent ones:

The fear of dying. Although some people die from complications of some of the rheumatic diseases, the vast majority do not. This is one of those fears you should relegate to Mark Twain's comment that "I have had many fears in my life, and most of them did not happen." If you are a parent of young children, it is important that you let them know that you are not dying. Sometimes in our own anxiety we forget just how frightened our children are when we are ill. If we don't give them any information, they usually imagine the very worst case. Discuss the disease with them in age-appropriate ways. If they are old enough to understand, let them go with you to the doctor and ask them to help with your exercises and to remind you to take your medications.

The fear of being dependent on others. No one of us wants to have to be dependent on other people. This is one of those fears that should positively motivate us to actively pursue physical therapy, good nutrition, and the other means we are discussing to help you maintain your independence. But at various times in our lives most of us will be dependent on others. If you find that you have to depend on others for help, you will have to evaluate your situation. By all means, try to keep an upbeat attitude. It's a tough situation, but remember that most people are happy to lend a helping hand—unless of course you are a real Scrooge! Keep a smile on your face. Be grateful for their help, and let your supporters know frequently that you are grateful.

The fear of medications. I presume that we all know that every medication will have some side effect. To eliminate your fear regarding medicines, you need to educate yourself regarding good benefits versus bad side effects. Ask your physician to explain just exactly what you should expect from the medications. Remember that it is *your* body. Ultimately, what risks are you willing to take to control your arthritis? We each have a different tolerance for pain, so only you can answer that question.

The fear of the unknown. When we are operating out of ignorance, we usually imagine the very worst possible scenarios. It is up to you to ask questions, to educate yourself about the disease, and to move from the unknown to the known.

Each of you can probably enlarge and expand this list, based on what is happening in your life. Illness does create fears. Discuss them with friends and family members. Force them out into the bright daylight. That alone will help put them into perspective. Seek out other people with arthritis and see if they have had the same fears. You may be surprised. And people who have had arthritis for some time will be able to give you some creative tips on overcoming those fears. Some fears are indeed realistic and need to be addressed up front. But fear can cause paralysis in our behavior. In order to achieve our life goals we must overcome our fears, realistic or otherwise.

The pain, chronicity, and unpredictability of arthritis can also produce a lot of anger, anger that we may not even understand. Unfortunately, when we are angry, we usually lash out at those closest to us. Be careful! Don't alienate those who care the most. Anger is a normal reaction to an unfair situation. "Why should I be the one with arthritis?" you may ask. Be assured that there is nothing fair about that fact! But don't let arthritis destroy your most important relationships. Find creative ways to vent your anger other than screaming, blaming others, or withdrawing. Exercise, get in the shower and have a good cry, write about your anger, throw a pillow, turn the radio up really loud, imagine having a terrific turkey dinner. If all this doesn't work, get professional help. Anger is normal, but you need to keep it under control in order to control your arthritis.

If I'm the Leader, Why Can't I Plan Simple Things?

Aside from the obvious fact of being in pain, there are many really aggravating, irritating things about arthritis. At times it is an "invisible" disease. You may look the same but you just can't get out of bed. You may be getting ready for an appointment and you become extremely fatigued. You may have planned a wonderful vacation and all of a sudden you are in a "flare." All your joints hurt and you can't possibly go.

Inability to plan even simple daily activities leads to major frustration. You are disappointed, your friends and family are disappointed, or your employer is disappointed. When this happens, and it probably will with arthritis, you need to look at your life and try to observe if some symptoms are created by certain activities. Perhaps your life-style produces a lot of stress. The solutions may be as simple as resting beforehand, rearranging medications, or having alternate plans. Letting people know ahead of time that you may not be able to make it, and encouraging them to continue without you, will alleviate some of the other people's frustration. In severe cases, after you have exhausted all the possibilities of controlling your arthritis, you may have to consider a career change—and that need not be the end of the world.

Acceptance as a Beginning

When my daughter was 15 years old and had been battling severe rheumatoid arthritis for about four years, she made a comment that I will never forget. Elizabeth had begun taking gold injections, and many people had told me that they were very painful. One woman said that she would rather have the pain of the arthritis than take those injections. Yet each time we went to Earl Brewer's office for an injection, my daughter never even blinked an eye. On several occasions I asked if the shots were painful, a question which Elizabeth never fully answered. Finally one day, while waiting for the elevator, I asked her again. Elizabeth looked at me with a fierce determination and said, "Don't you know, Mom, that what is pain for other people is different for me? I have accepted the fact that I have arthritis. I have to accept the pain that it brings and incorporate it into my life or it will destroy me. I have more important things to do with my life than worry about this pain." Her observations helped me to get past some of the pain I was having and get on with my life, too. Profound words from a very young lady!

The sooner you accept the fact that you have arthritis, the sooner you will be able to begin the process of getting on with your life. Certainly there is a period of grieving, but don't let that grief dominate your life for very long. It is the only life you have. Please make the very best of it!

In the next chapter we will look at the different members of your health team and what you should expect from each one.

9

Building a Coordinated Team

Life is definitely becoming more complicated. Technology is improving at a sometimes alarming rate. It is difficult, if not impossible, to keep up with the expanding knowledge in many areas. Medicine is one of the most rapidly changing fields, and it is becoming more and more specialized. The amiable family doctor who held your hand and explained what problem you were facing is a thing of the past. It is now impossible for one person to have an understanding of every aspect of medicine and every illness to which we are susceptible. Even within a specialized area, such as rheumatology, it is difficult for a physician to have a complete understanding of the more than a hundred types of rheumatic diseases.

In the past, medical science had quick, immediate responses to acute care problems. If an appendix is inflamed, take it out. If a leg is broken, splint it. But now, people are living longer, and there will be a greater need to treat the illnesses of aging, arthritis being one of the most dominant. Medicine has to change from a crisis care to a chronic care function. And because rheumatic diseases are chronic and ongoing, the need for education becomes imperative, and the relationship between physician and patient becomes much different. Education requires time and effort on the part of many people. A physician may not be knowledgeable in the field of physical therapy, for example. He may not know a lot about relaxation techniques to help you with chronic pain and stress reduction. You may also need the help of a podiatrist, a hand specialist, an occupational therapist, or any number of other health care specialists. Your primary care physician should be able to refer you to these people.

We participate in team efforts throughout our lives. What thoughts come to mind when you hear the word *team*? *Working together. All for one. Shoulder to shoulder. Cover all the bases. A strong offensive.* These are the exact phrases that should apply to your health team. When you think about building a team to help you reach your goal of living a terrific life, remember that it must start with *you!* You have to decide that you will not be defeated by this disease, that you will have control of your own life. You have to set your own personal goals. What limitations are you *not* willing to accept, and how are you going to overcome those limitations? Let's look at the different members of your team and how you can work with each one.

The Physician

There are many types of doctors who treat arthritis. A family practitioner is trained to take care of a variety of health care problems. He may take care of your child's infected tonsils and your grandmother's osteoarthritis. An internist is also qualified to treat many illnesses, including arthritis. However, if you have a really serious, debilitating type of arthritis, it would be in your best interest to find a good rheumatologist, an internal medicine doctor with special training in arthritis. There are also pediatric rheumatologists who specialize in children. If you have degenerative joint disorders, you will need to see a rheumatologist, and the earlier the better. There needs to be close collaboration between your primary care physician, rheumatologist, and the orthopedist. They will evaluate any structural defects, perform reconstructive surgery if needed, and with your input decide if joint replacement will help you.

For problems related to the feet, your doctor will probably refer you to a podiatrist. This foot specialist will examine your feet, check the wear patterns on your shoes, and perhaps recommend a specific type of footwear with special cushioning to reduce pressure. There are many devices that help ease painful nails, bunion deformities, hammertoes, and metatarsal depressions to make your life more comfortable. Major foot surgery is usually handled by an orthopedic surgeon.

Whichever types of doctors you choose, understand that you are the consumer, and that you are the one paying the bills. The quality of your life is in the balance, and you need not settle for anything less than excellence. Be sure that the doctor you choose is doing more than just prescribing medicine. His ability to explain and educate is very important in maximizing your efforts. While some people prefer to let the physician take control and don't want to know all the details, others want to be educated about the disease in order to make their own decisions. You need to find a doctor that suits your needs and your personality.

Seek out people you respect, whether it is a physician or a

good friend, and ask for their opinions and recommendations. Make sure the doctor is board certified in their specialty by calling the local medical society. However, even if a doctor is well trained but cannot impart his or her knowledge in a useful, compassionate manner, it won't help you. One of the most important qualities to look for is mutual respect. The treatment of arthritis is usually a long-term proposition. You will probably see more of your physician than you would like, so a good working relationship is really important. At some point you may need to get a second opinion for a variety of reasons, not the least of which is your peace of mind. A good doctor will not mind if you seek another opinion.

You need to be able to ask all the questions that are on your mind. Most people are intimidated by going to the doctor. The very thought conjures up an assortment of unpleasant feelings. You are undressed, you are poked, you are asked very personal questions. It is not fun, yet you need answers, you need direction. A little planning will go a long way. When a question occurs to you, write it down. Make a list. Be ready to ask questions as well as answer them. Good communication skills are a must, and good communication is complicated by the very fact that you are ill and probably in an emotional state, especially when you are first diagnosed. This is an extremely trying time, and while you try to absorb exactly what it means to have arthritis, you will not be terribly receptive to new information, even though it is important to your well-being. At some point you will probably find yourself asking the same questions you asked earlier. A well-organized physician will give you written materials to take home and read at your leisure.

If a doctor is using language that you don't understand, let him or her know. A recent study indicated that physicians, on the average, interrupted patients at about 18-second intervals. If you find that happening, you can be reasonably sure that the doctor is probably not listening to you. She or he is thinking about the next question for you, or analyzing something else. Don't let this happen. Just say, "Time out!" Tell the doctor you have a question, or an observation, or that you need help with this problem. On the other hand, part of the problem can often be attributed to the patient. Time is always a pressure in the day of a busy physician. Organize your questions and ask the most important ones first. Many people are afraid of bad news, so they save their more serious questions for last. By the time they get around to asking "the big one," there is another patient anxiously waiting to see the doctor, and you may not receive the complete information you need.

Arthritis is a difficult disease to treat. Each person responds in a different way to the news that he or she has the disease. Each person's body reacts differently to the various medications used to treat arthritis. Remember that it can be equally frustrating for the doctor if he or she is unable to control your symptoms. And each person makes decisions about just how much effort to put into fighting the disease. Proper treatment is a real juggling act, and in our high-tech world we often want an instant cure, a "magic pill." It doesn't exist. The sooner we all make up our minds that the road will be a twisting one, the sooner we will be successful in this effort. It is important that you feel that your doctor is your advocate and is serious about helping you along that road.

The Nurse

In a physician's office the nurse may play many different roles. She will play a large part in the ongoing education of the patient and the patient's family. In most settings it is easier to talk to the nurse and ask her to explain or clarify what the doctor told you. Frequently, the nurse will be sensitive to comments and observations that the doctor might have missed. A good nurse will know how to evaluate these casual comments and translate them into proper care for you.

Questions you may have about the side effects of medication can usually be answered by the nurse, or if she doesn't know the answer, she has better access to the doctor. Some nurses are trained in the field of rheumatology and can be of invaluable help in assessing many different aspects of the disease, including helping with modifications in the home, office, or perhaps school setting to make your life a little easier. A good nurse will become a counselor, a friend, and an advocate for you. The course of your arthritis will depend in great part on the coordination of care by many different health professionals, but the nurse is one of your most important contacts.

The Physical Therapist

Physical therapy has to be one of the most important aspects in the treatment of arthritis. While the physician attempts to control inflammation and damage to joints through medication, the physical therapist will help you maintain your mobility needed for daily activities—getting in and out of bed, getting in and out of chairs, safely navigating the bath, walking and climbing stairs safely. The therapist can evaluate your individual needs and show you new ways to do the things we all take for granted. We are talking about living life as normally as possible. There will be an initial evaluation by the physical therapist of how much the arthritis is affecting your body, where it is active, how many joints are involved, and what limitations you are having. Based on these observations, a treatment plan will be organized. The goal is to keep you as active and productive as possible.

Pain relief comes in many forms, from water therapy to relaxation techniques to biofeedback. The therapist can explain exactly what heat and cold will do to joints, and which of these might help you. He or she will also recommend range-of-motion exercises based upon the initial evaluation, and then periodically reassess them as your needs change. Don't underestimate the importance of these exercises. When you hear the phrase *physical therapy,* don't be intimidated. You will be taught very simple, straightforward exercises aimed at certain problem joints. There is nothing mysterious about them, but the results can be very dramatic.

We are definitely a goal-oriented society, one that has always stressed achievement and accomplishment. We often feel guilty about not being constantly on the go. You may be surprised to hear the therapist recommend rest as part of your treatment. It is part of pacing yourself. What good is it to go into overdrive and then spend days in bed? Be kind to your body and listen to your body. The physical therapist can teach you this new skill of being kind to your body.

The Occupational Therapist

"Occupational therapist" is somewhat misleading. The "occupational" part does not refer necessarily to work in the usual sense of the word. This important team member helps you to be independent and sees to it that you are functioning to the very best of your ability in every daily setting, wherever you may be, whether at work, at home, or in recreational activities. All qualified occupational therapists should be registered with the American Occupational Therapy Association.

The occupational therapist knows all sorts of methods and devices to use to help you go about your daily routine while conserving energy and minimizing damage to joints. She or he will design and fit any splints or other devices you might need to support or protect weakened joints and to help prevent certain deformities. With the occupational therapist's guidance, you can learn new ways of doing traditional things. By simplifying tasks, organizing your work in one area, using devices that improve efficiency, and learning how to adapt your environment, you can make your life easier.

Occupational therapists are employed in hospital settings, rehabilitation centers, and agencies such as the Visiting Nurses' Association.

The Social Worker

A social worker can help you with social and emotional concerns regarding your arthritis. They are knowledgeable about community resources that can assist you. You will find social workers in hospitals, mental health clinics, and church-related counseling services. They can help you through the maze of bureaucratic agencies that were established to assist people with disabilities, including the Social Security Administration and the various state agencies. Social workers have an undergraduate degree or a master's degree (M.S.W.). The letters A.C.S.W. (Academy of Certified Social Workers) after the person's name indicate that the social worker has passed a written examination and has at least two years of experience in the field. Social workers have training in counseling with individuals and families, and sometimes groups. Not all are informed about the problems related to arthritis. Your physician should know which social worker is knowledgeable about the problems you might be facing or inform the social worker about particular problems facing arthritis patients.

If you are unable to continue in your usual employment, social workers can guide you to job counselors in your state, find aid to help you retrain for another vocation or help you find other employment through your state's Department of Vocational Rehabilitation. The social worker can help determine just what benefits you may be eligible for, such as Social Security, Disability, Supplemental Security Income (SSI), or Aid to Families with Dependent Children (AFDC).

A good social worker knows the ins and outs of Medicare and Medicaid programs. These programs are part of a network including all sorts of supplemental home care (visiting nurses, physical therapists, transportation, meal services, recreational activities, and psychological care). In families with children who have arthritis, the social worker can intervene with the school to help prevent problems in that area. Laws have been passed to protect the rights of children in the school and a social worker should be knowledgeable about those ever-changing laws. The worker can also help the family members understand the psychological problems they may be facing. This person is a veritable font of information and help!

The Nutritionist

Most people may not eat a balanced, healthy diet. But if you have arthritis, the disease will have an effect on how you eat or don't eat, and the medications used to control the disease will have an impact on how your body processes the nutrients in the foods you do eat. Nutrition is always an important part of taking care of yourself, but now it becomes a medically important topic. The nutritionist is there to advise you about the way foods interact, how the drugs impact your system, and the part that vitamins play in your particular problem. The old saying "You are what you eat" could well be changed to "You feel as well as what you eat."

Nutrition has been sorely neglected in the medical school curriculum, so your doctor might not have a great deal of knowledge about nutrition. If you feel you need help in this area, ask your doctor if he knows of a good nutritionist, or ask friends and neighbors. Or take matters into your own hands and look through the Yellow Pages.

The Psychologist or Psychiatrist

Yes, indeed, life is difficult! Many people seek help in the form of psychological counseling for one reason or another. As stated before, the struggle with arthritis is not just a physical one but an emotional one as well. A professional counselor can help you put your problems with arthritis in perspective. This person is there to help you understand the impact your mind has on your disease, and it is major. A really good counselor will teach you how to use the power of the mind to your advantage. Researchers continue to be amazed at the tremendous power the mind has over the body.

It has been demonstrated that humor does many beneficial things to the body. Relaxation techniques are helping many people cope with chronic pain and stress. The psychologist or psychiatrist can help you maximize all the tools that are housed in your head in order for you to live the best life possible.

The psychologist can help you understand the dynamics of your relationships with other people. Arthritis can dramatically affect how you interact with others. If you develop a negative self-image, you will project that image to the world. The messages you receive in turn will also be negative. If arthritis is a fact in your life, it is better to accept that fact. And attitudes are more important than facts! How you attack the problem of arthritis will have a tremendous impact on how arthritis will attack your life. It is within your power to decide how arthritis will affect your daily life, and how it will affect your relationships with others.

If your physician is unable to refer you to a specific health professional, call your local chapter of the Arthritis Foundation and ask for their help. They will have a directory of members of the Arthritis Health Professionals Association.

I would like to be able to give you guidelines regarding how to pay for all the services you will need, what insurance to look for, which services insurance companies will pay for. I was recently in Houston visiting my daughter, who had just passed the Texas bar examination. Virginia was trying to understand an insurance policy. She became more and more exasperated, and asked if I could interpret the policy for her. I looked at her with a great deal of sympathy and said, "If you, a new lawyer, cannot read that thing, how do you think the average citizen, like me, could understand it?"

Try to find an honest agent who represents several companies. Ask questions pertinent to your problems. Realize that if you change jobs and have to find a new insurance company, and you have been diagnosed with arthritis, you are going to hear the phrase *pre-existing condition*. It will be difficult to find a company that will cover your condition. If you are eligible for Medicare or Medicaid, some of the services prescribed by your physician will be covered, at least partially.

The best news is that you don't have to tackle the problem alone. The people described in this chapter are just a few of the resources available to help you. Use them!

10

Medications

Medicines play an important role in your coordinated, comprehensive treatment program. As a rule, though, medicines for people with arthritis help but as yet don't cure. We can do our best to get rid of swelling, pain, redness, and tenderness of joints, improve joint motion, and reduce inflammation in other organs of the body such as the heart, eyes, and kidneys, but there's no "penicillin" to cure chronic arthritis.

Great progress has been made in developing anti–inflammatory or antiarthritis medicines that reduce pain and tenderness. Except for aspirin, most medications have come to market only in the past 20 or 30 years. Many physicians feel that we see far fewer people with terrible deformities as a result of using such medicines, but it is difficult to say for sure that this improved outlook is due to the medicine alone rather than a whole treatment program. Whatever the case, the relief of pain and swelling by one or more of these anti-inflammatory drugs allows you to begin an active, total program. Without significant relief of pain, all physical therapy programs are either hampered or just not possible. Aggressive treatment with the newer available medicines has resulted in less inflammation; and your strength, endurance, and joint motion are many times better than in the old days when people with arthritis were put to bed for months or years.

The immediate goal of drug therapy, therefore, is to relieve pain and swelling as soon as possible. The long-range goal is to alter the progress of the disease itself and its destruction of bone, cartilage, and soft tissues such as muscles, tendons, and joint capsules.

The subject of drugs and pregnancy is sufficiently complex that we are covering it in chapter 19, which is devoted to what happens to arthritis sufferers when they are pregnant.

Categories of Medicines

Two broad groups of drugs are used to treat people with arthritis: first-line nonsteroidal anti-inflammatory drugs (NSAIDs) and second-line drugs. The NSAIDs are always used first because they are usually safer, and if they fail to provide satisfactory relief, second-line drugs are *added* to the NSAIDs depending on the kind of arthritis that you have. We'll be discussing these drugs later on in this chapter.

The NSAIDs frequently used are aspirin, ibuprofen (Advil, Nuprin, Motrin, Rufen), Tolectin, Naprosyn, Orudis, Indocin, Feldene, Voltaren, Nalfon, Relafen, and Clinoril. Cortisone and its derivatives are in a class by themselves. The most important second-line drugs to know about are methotrexate, gold, d-penicillamine, hydroxychloroquine, sulfasalazine, and cytotoxic medicines.

There are also unconventional medicines that you may receive from helpful, well-meaning friends, people on the street, and relatives. Unfortunately, in any chronic arthritis of unknown cause, there have been any number of copper bracelets, herbs, medicines, devices, and foods that have helped people feel better for a little while. The problem with these is that arthritis is so variable that complete or partial relief of pain or swelling of joints may happen for no apparent reason at any time. An unconventional medicine that is taken at the same time that spontaneous improvement occurs may mistakenly get credit for the improvement.

At least 8 out of 10 people will try some unconventional treatment, usually one that's harmless but a waste of time and money. If you are tempted, ask your doctor about this so-called miracle cure. There is always a new magic cure from Mexico or Canada, and oddly enough, each "cure" has a half life of two or three years. The important thing to remember is not to harm yourself with a risky fad, or worse, to deny yourself proper treatment for some off-the-wall idea.

General Rules About Taking Medicine

One reason that so many medicines are manufactured for people with arthritis is that individuals respond differently to different medicines. A medicine that helps one person may not help another. Similarly, a medicine may cause unpleasant or even dangerous side effects in someone at some time, but not for you.

You and your doctor must weigh how much good a medicine can do against how bad its side effects may be in deciding whether to start or continue it. If a medicine helps you, and produces no bad side effects, it's immaterial whether it's dangerous to another person. If it is safe for you, this is the best measure of your decision. This is why the prescribed dose usually starts low, then increases to a level that either helps the arthritis or causes unsatisfactory side effects. Nor do you need to despair if unpleasant side effects occur; the dose can be reduced, and hopefully the side effect should disappear.

Additionally, the time required for a new medicine or an increased dose of an old medicine to effect improvement may be weeks or even months before further change is considered. This is why follow-ups to check for adverse effects of a drug are vital. When the physician or nurse asks you to come in for a safety check on the medicine, pay attention and do it; it's not just another way to pad the bill. Often a blood count, urinalysis, or a liver function test is required at intervals of days, weeks, or months depending on the drug and its effect on you, so get these done if your doctor orders them.

Inform yourself of the action of a drug. A few drugs are strictly analgesic, that is, they help pain only. Acetaminophen (Tylenol) is useful for headaches and the aches and pains of arthritis. Medicines containing narcotics are analgesics also. Anti-inflammatory drugs such as NSAIDs reduce inflammation and help pain by reducing swelling.

Finally, you should inquire of your doctor or nurse when you begin a new medicine about any drug interactions with other medicines you may be taking. Ask also if there are any special instructions relating to the absorption of the medicine. For example, is it important to take it between meals, or right at bedtime? Ask the druggist who fills the prescription if she has substituted a generic drug, and if so, what are the differences?

If You Experience Adverse Side Effects

The usual adverse reactions to drugs are fairly straightforward and can be monitored to ensure safety. Fewer than 1 person in 20 has to stop a medicine because of bad side effects; aspirin is an exception with 1 in 6 taken off this drug. Anemia, along with a loss of white blood cells or platelets, can occur with almost any arthritis drug. The kidney or the liver can also be injured. A blood count, urinalysis, and liver function test are the usual tests done to check on the most frequent side effects of drugs, though many adverse effects do not require a test to be detected. Diarrhea and skin rashes are frequent signs of adverse effects, for example.

If a side effect is not serious, ignore it if the medicine is helping. If it is serious, then you and the doctor will have to weigh how much good the medicine is doing against how much injury the adverse effect is causing. For example, many people get a rash from medicines. If the rash is mild and the medicine is helping, you might want to continue the drug since its overall effect is positive.

It is important to distinguish between an allergy and other adverse effects. Allergy to any of these drugs occurs in less than 1 in 100 people. The two chief ways that allergic reactions occur are in the skin with hives or itching, or asthma-like symptoms with difficulty breathing. This is different from local irritation of the intestinal tract, for example.

Remember that many things can play a role in side effects, and so you need to be certain that a side effect is due to the medicine. Your doctor will usually ask you to stop the medicine for a week or longer to see if the rash or blood in the urine disappears. If it does, he or she will ask you to restart the drug. Many times, strangely enough, the rash or blood in the urine does not recur, and therefore wasn't due to the medicine. You see how important it is not only to stop the medicine but to rechallenge the body to be sure a drug side effect has occurred.

When a New Medicine Is Added

When the physician and you decide that a new medicine is needed, several steps usually occur. The physician or educator will explain how the medicine is thought to work, what dose to take, and the possible side effects. You will be directed to take a low dose at first. You will also be asked to return in one to two weeks for a safety check. You will be asked about any side effects such as diarrhea, abdominal pain, headaches, blurred vision, or drowsiness. Most medicines don't take effect so quickly, and improvement isn't expected by this initial checkup. If you feel better, consider yourself lucky.

The next safety check and office visit will probably be a month or two later. In the case of NSAIDs, continuation for at least two and maybe three months is necessary to be reasonably sure that the drug will or will not work. In the case of the slower-acting drugs such as gold, a six-month trial is necessary before giving up. *Patience is the hardest lesson to learn, especially when you are stiff and hurting.*

During my 30 years of caring for people with arthritis, the most frequent reason for a referral from other doctors was the patient's complaint that none of the medicines was effective any longer. However, 9 times out of 10 the medicines had not been given sufficient time to work. Remember: If you badger your doctor to change medicines every few weeks and don't give them a chance to work, you'll never find a medicine that helps you!

When the Medicine Quits Working

Medicines do sometimes quit working. There's nothing more distressing than when aspirin, some other NSAID, or gold controls the pain and swelling satisfactorily for months or years and then suddenly stops being effective. Sometimes this occurs because the druggist substituted a generic drug from another company. Usually, however, the medicine just stops working. We call this *tachyphylaxis*, and it is not your fault. When tachyphylaxis occurs, your doctor may stop the medicine and start another. Sometimes increasing the dose helps, but then adverse effects can occur. Usually another medicine is necessary. The failed medicine can be prescribed again months or years later and be effective. It's almost as if whatever suddenly blocked the effectiveness has disappeared—perhaps an antibody or immune response—but physicians don't yet have these answers.

NSAIDs

Many of the NSAIDs currently in use have similar qualities and are grouped together. Many doctors call them "me too" medications because they are so similar in action. They do not contain any cortisone or its derivativess, hence the term *nonsteroidal*. They suppress inflammation, meaning that they reduce swelling, pain, tenderness, and redness as well as improve motion, hence the term, *anti-inflammatory*. Their exact modes of action are not known, but they seem to inhibit parts of a chemical cycle in the body that causes inflammation.

NSAIDs are the initial treatment of choice for most kinds of arthritis. They offer the best and safest help in reducing swelling and pain in joints and in managing fever. They usually begin to help in terms of weeks, though you can expect releif from fever within hours. However, sometimes they have to be given for months before improvement is apparent. In general, several NSAIDs will be tried before second-line drugs are considered.

The best known NSAID is aspirin, which is the original and oldest NSAID, in use since the last century before the Food and Drug Administration (FDA) was formed. For this reason aspirin has always been an over-the-counter drug. The other NSAIDs are prescription drugs except ibuprofen (Advil, Nuprin, and others). Other NSAIDs must be approved by the FDA for use in people with arthritis. Acetaminophen (Tylenol and others) is considered a painkiller only and is also sold over the counter.

How NSAIDs are administered. All NSAIDs are administered by mouth, although aspirin is sometimes given by suppository. In Europe suppositories are a popular way of administering NSAIDs because they reduce stomach pain and nausea, but they are less popular here because Americans are uncomfortable about administering drugs through the anus. Local irritation of the anal area is a possible side effect. At the moment there are no NSAID skin-patch preparations, though the idea is good because skin patches allow even absorption. This will probably occur sometime in the future.

The NSAIDs differ markedly in how often they must be given. The most commonly used NSAIDs—aspirin and the ibuprofen drugs—have short blood-level times of a few hours. They must be given at least three times or four times daily. Others such as Naproxen (Naprosyn) have longer blood-level times of 12 to 14 hours after a dose and need to be given only two times daily. One drug, Feldene, has a half life of greater than one day and can be given once daily.

Should NSAIDs be given with meals or between meals? Well, the drug level is higher if taken on an empty stomach, but stomach pain and nausea are also more frequent. Also, while a better drug level will be attained with between-meal dosage, it's easier for most people to remember to take the medicine at mealtimes. The specific time of day that medicine is given also matters. Most NSAIDs provide better results if given in higher doses at bedtime and in lower doses during the day. But with the short-acting medicines, daytime doses are just as necessary.

In short, if your medication is to be taken two times daily, take it at breakfast and at bedtime with a little food or milk. When medication once a day is possible, bedtime may be better. Also, when nausea is a problem, giving the evening dose at bedtime is better because the nausea occurs when you are asleep. No matter what they tell you, most NSAIDs keep fever down for no more than five hours regardless of the half life of the medicine in the blood.

A definite concern to everyone is: how long can NSAIDs be safely given? As far as anyone knows, they can be given for many years with no long-term dangers.

What type of relief to expect. NSAIDs have three main uses: to reduce swelling and inflammation, relieve pain, and reduce fever. NSAIDs improve fever the fastest. Reduction in an hour is frequent, though with JRA several hours may be necessary to control the high fever. Reducing pain in the joint is the next improvement, followed by reduced stiffness, reduced swelling and tenderness, and improvement of motion. Overall improvement in the joints can occur in a few days' time, but usually weeks and sometimes months can pass before noticeable improvement occurs. In fact, NSAIDs have allowed some patients to cut back on their intake of cortisone.

Until a few years ago, aspirin was the universal drug of choice for arthritis. However, since other NSAIDs have fewer side effects, the use of aspirin has been reduced. Also, because of Reye's syndrome, a terrible disease that affects the liver and brain of young children, its use has been severely restricted. Aspirin also causes liver function abnormalities in 1 in 6 children.

In the *Physician's Desk Reference* there are more than 30 brands of NSAIDs listed that are on the market now, with perhaps 20 or more in the process of approval by the FDA. Part of the reason, of course, is the competitive spirit of our free economy, but another reason is that not everyone responds to a particular NSAID; therefore, several different ones are necessary. Some NSAIDs represent attempts to improve side effects such as headaches, drowsiness, or stomach pain and ulcers. Other NSAIDs can be given fewer times daily to increase compliance as mentioned.

When all things are considered, the treatment effects are the same with all of the NSAIDs. No single one is clearly better than another. No single one has side effects that are absent in the others. The difference is that each person responds differently to each drug, and what helps one person will not help another. In addition, if one drug quits working, we need to be able to try another.

Every physician has a favorite NSAID that seems to work best for his or her patient. By using only a few NSAIDs the doctor is more familiar with the dosage variations and usual side effects; this frequently results in better treatment than if she or he uses many NSAIDs on an infrequent basis and is not as familiar with individual variations of each one.

In general, NSAIDs should be given for one month before changing to another. There is a 50 percent chance that the first NSAID will be effective, and therefore a 50 percent chance for subsequent trials of different NSAIDs. It usually takes a trial of two or three NSAIDs before a safe and effective one is found. Usually a second-line drug is considered when two or three NSAIDs have been unsuccessful. If destructive arthritis appears or the disease worsens appreciably, second-line drugs are usually added.

Possible side effects of NSAIDs. The list of adverse effects of NSAIDs is long, but the major problems are few. The intestinal tract heads the list with nausea, abdominal pain, vomiting, and diarrhea. Anemia and blood or protein in the urine are next in frequency. Headache or drowsiness is infrequent. Changes in liver function frequently occur in children but not in adults who use aspirin, but changes in liver function are rare in children using the other NSAIDs.

About 5 percent of people receiving NSAIDs will have to discontinue them because of unacceptable side effects, particularly intestinal problems or anemia. A particular problem with aspirin is hemorrhaging in the intestinal tract in one in a hundred people taking aspirin.

The liver function tests used most often, called transaminase tests, monitor the enzymes the liver uses to break down chemicals in the body. The tests go by many names, but two are the SGOT and SGPT. They are done a few weeks after starting a new NSAID and every few months for a while to be sure that a particular medication is not injuring the liver. When the tests show results that are greater than two or three times normal, the doctor will usually tell you to stop the medicine and later may try to lower the daily dose to see if a lower dose will still help the arthritis and not cause the liver to function abnormally. Again, it's always a battle to find a medicine that helps the arthritis enough yet has minimal side effects.

NSAIDs cause anemia in 2 or 3 percent of people, though it's difficult to know whether the anemia is due to the arthritis or the medicine. Again, the usual sequence for a doctor to follow is to stop the medicine for a week or longer in order to see whether the blood count increases. The anemia can last for months or longer. The reason for the prolonged anemia is that the medication has depressed the blood-forming organs—the bone marrow.

You should pay attention to requests for a blood count safety check.

Urinalysis tests are used to check for blood or protein. When either is present in significant amounts in the urine specimen, it usually means that injury to the kidney has occurred. Aspirin rarely causes this type of problem; the injury more often occurs with one of the other NSAIDs. The same rules of stopping the drug, as mentioned above, apply here also.

Second-line Drugs

When NSAIDs alone do not help inflammation and pain sufficiently, other antirheumatic drugs are usually added for people with inflammatory types of arthritis. Rheumatoid arthritis is the main condition that requires additional therapy. Cortisone is rapid in action and in its own class. Methotrexate is a rapidly acting and effective second-line drug used in people with significant RA who have been unresponsive to NSAIDs. Unlike these, several other of the second-line drugs take months to have an effect and so are termed *slower-acting antirheumatic drugs.* Included in this group are gold, d-penicillamine, and hydroxychloroquine. Gold is the most effective drug of this group and works best in the injectable form. All of them are probably anti-inflammatory in some manner.

Cortisone

Cortisone or its better-known derivative, prednisone, came on the scene in the 1950s. Corticosteroids suppress the immune system to reduce inflammation. Initial doses are truly like a miracle. Within days the person suffering from severe and debilitating arthritis loses pain and stiffness and may even be able to run. That's pretty heady stuff if you've been lying in bed miserable with pain. The trouble is that the initial dosage will soon need to be increased to maintain the effect. Like hard drugs, cortisone takes more and more to satisfy, and eventually not only do bad effects occur, but the good effect doesn't last. Even worse, when the dose is reduced, the pain and swelling come back with a vengeance. In children, cortisone stops or slows normal growth and can dwarf a child.

Most physicians try to use cortisone as a last resort or in severe situations, since it is clearly the most effective anti-inflammatory medicine, but the side effects make us think carefully before using it. When necessary, however, it is the best and most effective medicine in our cabinet of drugs, and many people with RA and other inflammatory diseases take low doses of steroids with good results and little toxicity.

By the way, don't confuse corticosteroids with the male-hormone "steroids" mentioned in the press in connection with athletes who take them to increase their strength. The two are completely different in that those steroids are the male hormone, not cortisone.

How corticosteroids are given. Steroids are given by mouth or injected into the muscle or the veins if necessary. Tablets and liquids are used in most situations. Injections are usually reserved for hospital care. Prednisone is the main steroid used in the United States. Steroid eye drops are the usual treatment of choice for iritis.

What type of relief to expect with cortisone. When a person with RA is slipping fast, nothing improves the disease better than steroids, which often quickly control fever, severe pain and swelling in the joints, and inflammation in the eyes. Steroids initially provide a general sense of well-being or euphoria that helps in relieving pain enough to get the sufferer moving again. Eventually, however, the drug quits working, and side effects occur. With an enormous amount of effort, the dose can be slowly reduced over months and months a little bit at a time until it is low enough to be safe. When tolerated by the body with no serious side effects, steroids are given in small doses for years with success.

Possible side effects. It's important to say at the outset that when steroids are given for only a month or two, the serious side effects discussed here do not usually occur. Even in people who require large doses to control incapacitating RA for months or years, many of the side effects will largely disappear after the medicine is stopped. So if steroids don't affect you adversely, it's the most useful medicine we have.

Fluid retention, or edema, is a serious side effect. A person taking large doses can blow up like a blimp and gain 10 to 20 pounds. Such a weight gain is not only unattractive but dangerous because excessive fluid in the body causes hypertension or high blood pressure. When the steroids are reduced or stopped, the high blood pressure goes away.

Steroids also cause a loss of calcium from the bones, or osteoporosis, which can lead to fractures of the back or other bones. Periodic X rays can reveal when osteoporosis is excessive. It can also be measured by a densitometer, an electronic device that measures the density of bone. Usually the severity of disease must be weighed against the loss of calcium in deciding whether to continue steroids for a long period of time.

Cataracts can occur in people using long-term cortisone. "Masking" of infections can also be a problem. This occurs when steroids make you feel better if you have bronchitis or some other infection that normally makes you feel terrible. You are deceived and think that the illness is not a big deal when it is. Even though this is a definite problem, it rarely causes confusion when you are ill. If in doubt, check with your doctor.

Steroids also affect the skin, in that small blood vessels bleed with little or no trauma; this easy bruising is unsightly but not serious.

Some people experience emotional changes with steroids. Indeed, a good side effect is the euphoria that occurs at times. Unfortunately, behavior problems can occur also. All are reversed when the steroids are stopped.

While not a problem in adults, steroids retard growth in children. The dose required to inhibit growth varies in each child. In some children, large doses for weeks, months, or even years do not affect growth. In a few children, growth is completely stopped with only a milligram or two daily. When the medication is stopped, growth resumes in a few months, if the bones are still capable of growth. In children who have no apparent loss of the growth curve, there is no reason to worry.

Methotrexate

Methotrexate alters special chemical processes in the body that affect immune cells and is anti-inflammatory in action. It affects the metabolism of one of the vitamins, folic acid. Its precise way of helping arthritis is not known. It has been used in cancer treatment for many years. In the high doses required in cancer treatment, many side effects occur. Its use in RA originated when dermatologists found excellent results when it was given to people with psoriasis, whose arthritis was also greatly improved. In RA, very low doses are used weekly instead of daily, thereby reducing side effects.

How methotrexate is given. Methotrexate is usually given one day each week by mouth in one to three doses to reduce nausea. It can also be injected into the veins or muscles. It is important that laboratory tests of blood and urine be done every few weeks at first and then every few months later to check for side effects. Monthly liver function tests are a good idea also.

What type of relief to expect. Methotrexate is in a class by itself in the treatment of RA and JRA. It is also used in other rheumatic diseases such as polymyositis. In study after study of adults with severe or milder RA, methotrexate is clearly better than a placebo. In one study by Dr. Michael Weinblatt and associates of Boston, pain and tenderness improved in approximately 70 percent of RA patients and only 20 percent of placebo patients. Swelling of joints improved in over 60 percent of patients with RA and 20 percent of placebo patients.

In a recently completed cooperative study between the United States and Russia, 120 children with severe JRA from both countries received methotrexate for six months once a week. Over 70 percent improved greatly, while only 40 percent of the group that took NSAIDs alone improved. This is far better than any of the other drugs studied thus far. In some situations the improvement was startling.

Methotrexate is particularly useful because it allows steroids to be given in smaller doses, which reduces side effects. Many times it allows the steroid to be stopped completely. Another good feature is that the majority of people are still on methotrexate five years later. This is not true with the other second-line drugs.

Possible side effects. Unlike cortisone, methotrexate does not affect growth. The side effects are the same as those already mentioned with other antirheumatic drugs. Mouth ulcers, intestinal symptoms of nausea or upset stomach, and anemia occur occasionally. In the doses used, side effects have been minimal in study patients. Early in use there was considerable worry about liver damage, but further study shows that the risk in RA is low. Alcohol consumption is a risk factor for liver damage. Initially years ago, liver biopsies were done on all patients before methotrexate was administered and then a year or so later. This is no longer necessary. We know changes do occur in the liver but serious injury has not been a problem in people who do not abuse alcohol.

Methotrexate affects folic acid, a vitamin in the body, and a deficiency of folic acid can occur, causing anemia, mouth ulcers, or upset stomach. Some doctors give small doses of folic acid daily to prevent this.

We all worry about future side effects of any drug given, and methotrexate is no exception. Potential side effects include some reduction of sperm cells in men only while they are taking the medicine. It has no effect on function of the ovaries. Libido and sex drive are not affected. If taken during pregnancy, the fetus can be affected. For women of child-bearing potential, birth control is essential while taking methotrexate. It also can cause injury to the lungs, so smokers taking methotrexate should stop smoking; and as with any drug, serious allergic reactions can occur. However, in the doses used for rheumatic disease, this drug rarely causes serious problems, and fewer than 5 percent of people taking methotrexate have to stop because of side effects.

Gold

Gold, the precious metal, has been used in medicine for centuries. Gold therapy has been a mainstay in the treatment of RA since the 1920s. The drug acts to suppress inflammation of the joints in ways that are not clear despite many years of experience. Until methotrexate was found to be so effective and safe, gold was the most frequently used second-line drug in the United States and other parts of the world. The concern about methotrexate's side effects still make gold a major alternative.

How gold is given. Gold can be given orally or by injection. The usual way is to give gold by injection into the muscle weekly for four or five months. Maintenance injections are then given every two to four weeks indefinitely. Oral gold (Ridaura) may be given daily for an indefinite period of time.

What type of relief to expect. With gold treatment the first improvement is reduced morning stiffness, usually after two to four months of use. At four to six months joint swelling, pain, and tenderness begin to disappear. Gold does not help the fever of RA. If you are unable to tell whether you are better after six months of gold therapy, you and your doctor need to think about stopping the drug and trying something else.

Injectable gold is more effective than oral gold. Oral gold, however, is easier to take and has fewer side effects. When the oral gold is effective, it is preferable. Some doctors begin with oral gold for this reason. If in six months no improvement is apparent, injectable gold is given for six months. The response rate is about the same as NSAIDs: 50 percent. Remember that gold is added to the NSAID, not taken instead of the NSAID.

Possible side effects. About 10 percent of children and adults on gold will need to stop because of unacceptable side effects such as anemia, low white-blood-cell count, or liver-function-test abnormalities. The kidneys can be affected also. A drug rash can occur but is almost always mild and disappears when the dosage is reduced. Only rarely do serious adverse effects occur, and these changes are usually reversible if the medicine is stopped. It is most important to follow up with any lab safety checks your doctor requests.

Hydroxychloroquine (Plaquenil)

This interesting drug, which has long been a treatment for malaria, is thought to affect the body's immune system in dealing with arthritis. It was discovered as a treatment for arthritis when people taking it for malaria noticed improvement in their arthritis. In Russia and in a few areas in our country, Plaquenil is given to every person with RA from the first day of diagnosis. It is thought to relieve pain better and to reduce the number of flare-ups due to bad weather or illness.

In general, Plaquenil may be used as a last-resort medicine when others fail, and always with other drugs. Many arthritis doctors use it early in the course of the disease. When it helps, it really helps a lot. So it's worth trying as a far-down-the-list second-line drug. Remember, this is a general opinion, and your physician may think otherwise given your specific circumstance.

How plaquenil is given. It is given by mouth daily. Months and months of treatment are necessary to show effect.

What type of relief to expect. Plaquenil does seem to relieve pain in many people with RA. Proponents of its use believe that flare-ups are less frequent when the drug is used in conjunction with another medication. Like methotrexate, it can reduce the steroid dosage necessary in what is called a steroid-sparing effect.

Possible side effects. The side effects include the usual ones: low blood count, blood or protein in the urine, or abnormal liver function tests. Nausea and skin rashes can also occur. With high doses, injury to the back of the eye (retina) can occur, but usually the doses are low, and this does not happen. However, if you are taking Plaquenil, see your eye doctor every six to twelve months just to be safe.

D-penicillamine

D-penicillamine appears to act on the immune system in unknown ways to suppress arthritis. The drug was found to be helpful in adult RA patients by accident. It is a chelating agent, meaning that it binds heavy metals like gold and removes them from the body in patients with overdosage of gold. When it was used in treatment of gold overdosage in adult patients with rheumatoid arthritis, it relieved the arthritis.

This is considered to be a medication of last resort. On the other hand, some people with arthritis respond only to penicillamine and nothing else. It's always used with an NSAID and even other drugs such as steroids.

How d-penicillamine is given. D-penicillamine is given in tablet form daily. It must be given for several months before any effects are apparent.

What type of relief to expect. Studies by Dr. Ray Jaffe and many others showed improvement in joint swelling and pain in adults. The Pediatric Rheumatology Collaborative Study Group (PRCSG) conducted a controlled study of children with JRA, comparing d-penicillamine with NSAID alone and with hydroxychloroquine (Plaquenil). None of the three was better than the other. As is the case with Plaquenil, d-penicillamine can reduce the steroid dosage necessary. Some patients improve with d-penicillamine when NSAID alone does not help. For this reason, it remains one of the second-line drugs used when NSAIDs taken alone fail.

Possible side effects. Side effects are infrequent but can be serious. Milder side effects include loss of taste while taking the medicine as well as the usual effects already discussed in the blood, urine, and liver function tests. On rare occasions a muscular condition called myasthenia gravis can occur, which causes a weakness of muscles and is a serious illness.

Other Drugs

Several medicines comparable to the slower-acting antiarthritis drugs discussed above are not widely used in this country. Sulfasalazine (Azulfidine) is an anti-inflammatory drug used in Europe mainly for the relief of pain and arthritis. Observations by doctors and a few studies show mixed results in how helpful it is. In general, Azulfidine is prescribed only when the previously mentioned drugs are unsuccessful.

Cytotoxic drugs are cancer drugs that can and do cause malignancy. They also cause sterility and birth defects. These drugs are immunosuppressive, meaning that they lessen the body's defenses against infection. They also are more likely to cause serious injury to the blood, kidneys, and liver.

Future Drugs

New medicines and new approaches are the hope of the future. Currently, genetically produced antibodies or proteins that block cells or receptors on the surface of cells that do harm to the body are receiving intense interest. If these cells are successfully blocked in their actions by either destroying the cells or reducing their numbers, inflammation will be suppressed, and your arthritis will be somewhat alleviated. This use of special protein antibodies, called monoclonal antibodies, to inhibit or destroy "helper cells" in the body's immune system is a promising, experimental approach in the early stages.

Variations of this approach include adding a toxin or harmful substance to the monoclonal antibody to block specific chemicals and receptors on the surface of the T cells that cause inflammation. Two of the toxins are called anti-CD5 immunotoxin and Interleukin-2 toxin protein.

Another approach is to find a chemical similar to the destructive chemicals liberated by the T cells that damage the joints and cartilage. The "phony" chemical takes the place of the dangerous chemical, fooling the body, and no effect on the cells occurs, preventing joint destruction. Sound too good to be true? It is at the moment, but the possibility exists for productive knowledge to further help people with arthritis.

A Final Note

The basic lesson I hope you will take with you is that you will probably do best starting with NSAIDs. When NSAIDs are not enough, your doctor may consider second-line drugs in a sequence reflecting what he or she thinks will help and what kind of arthritis you have. Steroids are usually reserved for really bad problems. Methotrexate or gold is usually next in line. Other drugs are used when the top group fails to help any longer. You and your doctor will have to make the decisions of what to use, how much to give, and when to stop.

All of the medications are designed to improve motion and reduce pain, swelling, and inflammation. This allows you to do physical therapy and begin the road to improvement. Medicines are usually invaluable and enable the many faces of team care to be effective.

11

Exploring Alternative Therapies

The word *arthritis* has conjured up fear and anxiety in families for many generations. And those fears and anxieties have created some rather strange attempts to solve the problems of arthritis. Let's say you have come to the realization one day that you have arthritis. Your aunt Millie probably tried to treat your arthritis first, followed by your cousin Jane and probably more than a few friends. Maybe it was Aunt Millie who insisted that you wear that tight-fitting copper bracelet, even when your wrist turned green. When your symptoms didn't go away, she probably accused you of not wearing the bracelet all the time, right? It was your neighbor Mary who had her friend bring those terrible-tasting herbal teas to cure your pain. Good intentions all.

Unproven and Dangerous Remedies

Some folks even sit around in abandoned uranium mines in an effort to alleviate their arthritis symptoms. With radiation levels in the mines at 175 times the federally accepted standard, it might seem puzzling that people would be willing to take that kind of risk with unknown results. But that is the nature of this problem. Chronic pain can really make you desperate. When conventional treatments don't work, people will try just about anything—and a study indicates that about 94 percent of patients with arthritis will try one of these unproven remedies at least once.

If you're lucky, you have avoided some of the more dangerous "cures" for arthritis. Americans are spending some six billion dollars each year on useless "miracle cures" for arthritis. Because the diseases are so frustrating, and the pain so debilitating, it is understandable why people search for relief in just about any form. These unproven remedies range from rather innocuous ones to really hazardous ones.

Some of these treatments are harmless. Among the harmless ones are copper charms, herbal teas (provided they don't contain steroids), mineral waters, topical creams, and New Zealand green-lipped mussels. Others are potentially dangerous, with little scientific basis for the claims made on their behalf. For example, dimethyl sulfoxide (DMSO) is an industrial compound that has been touted as a relief for inflamed joints. While it may give temporary relief, it is unproven and may cause skin irritation and diarrhea. Other new treatments have not been thoroughly tested and their side effects are unknown. There have been claims that megadoses of certain vitamins will cure arthritis, but some vitamins can accumulate in the body to toxic levels. Snake venom and bee venom are also dangerous treatments because they may cause severe allergic reactions. Some drugs that are finding their way into this country contain unknown ingredients, among them steroids.

Many treatments may give you temporary relief simply because you believe they will. This is called the placebo effect. The mind is a truly powerful tool, and when we really focus on achieving a desired result, we may actually be able to gain relief, at least for a brief time. Also, arthritis is known for being up and down; you may feel good one day and miserable the next, and go into remissions for no apparent reason. People who spend time in a uranium mine might feel better only because they have simply removed themselves from everyday stress for a short time. This could also explain why people feel much better after going to one of those clinics that administer strange, unknown drugs. These clinics are almost always in beautiful, tropical settings, with warm climates. Just being in that environment would help *anyone* feel better.

Many of these unproven remedies will cost you quite a bit of money. My recommendation would be to save your money and take a friend out to lunch or open a savings account! Be logical when you are considering using any of these unproven remedies. Do they claim to cure arthritis? All 100 forms? (The types of arthritis are very different from one another and there would have to be many different cures.) Is it safe? Are the side effects known? (Every drug will have a side effect.) What scientific studies have been conducted to determine the effectiveness? Do these studies use the word *natural* to describe the remedy? (Snake venom is natural but it can be harmful.)

Look at the way the product is promoted. If a scientist finds a cure for one kind of arthritis it will not be touted as a cure-all, or based on a secret formula, or available through an 800 number. I guarantee that it will be on the front page of every newspaper and magazine in the country. It will be a cause for celebration. Snake oil salesmen have been around forever—don't fall for their smooth talk and dubious promises on cable television.

Alternative Remedies

Let's look at some of the constructive alternative ways in which people are finding relief from the everyday aggravations of arthritis. Being fit is by far the best answer to many of the problems facing people with arthritis, but these other methods might help you along the road. I would divide these techniques into physical and psychological approaches. First, let's examine some of the physical ways.

Acupuncture

Traditional Chinese medicine has practiced acupuncture for more than 2,500 years. Western scientists agree that acupuncture can work, although they cannot say why. Acupuncturists see the body as a bioelectric system with definite energy pathways. They believe there are 14 meridians, or energy channels, running through the body. Along those meridians are 361 acupuncture points. Some practitioners also identify 48 more points, with additional meridiens along the scalp. Others identify a set of needling points in the ear.

According to the accupuncture theory, when energy is disrupted along the meridians, pain and illness result. Needles are used to stimulate points along the channels, thereby balancing the flow and restoring health. There is some skepticism regarding the claims of acupuncture. However, respected medical journals such as the British journal *Lancet* have reported that these treatments may work well for certain patients with chronic back pain or painful joints. There is less proof for treating other ailments.

If you decide to try acupuncture for pain relief, and we are not specifically recommending it here, you should take care in choosing a practitioner. There is a problem of poorly trained and not very ethical acupuncturists. State laws vary with recognition of acupuncturists. You'll have to check with either a local medical society or the state board of medical examiners. In general, you're acting on faith alone.

Cleanliness is always of concern when there is an invasive procedure of any kind. In this age of AIDS it becomes a matter of life and death. The needles do pierce the skin, and you should allow only disposable needles to be used in acupuncture. As with all types of treatments, beware if there are exaggerated claims of "instant cures." All your questions should be answered clearly, and you should understand what will be done and what the treatment offers.

Chiropractic

A chiropractor treats diseases by manipulating the spine and other body structures, based on the belief that many diseases are caused by pressure, especially of the vertebrae, on nerves. Many people believe very strongly in this therapy because they do get relief from pain by the manipulations. Again, check the credentials of anyone administering this therapy. Make sure they are certified, and as always, beware of claims of instant cures. These are all methods of helping you cope with the pain of arthritis—they are not cures. Many rheumatologists and orthopedists are concerned because in chiropractic practice, more serious disease is not recognized, and a delay in treatment can result in further injury,

Massage Therapy

Massage is an ancient form of pain management and stress relief. The Chinese practiced it more than 3,000 years ago, and it has been used continually since then. Our lives today tend to be stress-filled, and massage is one way to help us relax our muscles and let our bodies be refreshed. As you read this you can probably identify areas of stress in your body. Are your shoulders tense? Is your neck stiff? Are you clenching your teeth? All this tension really aggravates the pain of arthritis. Massage is a way to help us relax and allow the blood to flow naturally through our bodies.

The types of massage range from stroking, either lightly or firmly, to increase blood flow, to compression, which is kneading or squeezing. There is also percussion, using the hands to strike the muscles. Some physical therapists use electric vibrators to massage the muscles.

One form of massage that is gaining in popularity is *shiatsu*. It is a Japanese technique that uses the fingers to apply pressure on the muscles. It can sometimes be uncomfortable when applied to sensitive areas. *Reflexology* is a variation on this theme, with pressure applied to specific areas of the soles of the feet. This theory holds that the muscles and organs of the body are affected by specific areas of the feet. It can be a very relaxing treatment.

Heat Treatment

Perhaps the oldest known treatment for arthritis is simply a hot bath. People have been going to resorts with hot mineral springs for centuries. Heat can be found in a hot bath, hot pack, or a heating pad. Another method of heat application is hot paraffin. Paraffin baths are simply heated containers filled with melted paraffin and wintergreen oil. Beauty salons use them as a hand treatment, but for arthritis sufferers these baths are a way to get deep heat to the small joints in the hands or feet. After dipping the hand a dozen times to coat it with hot paraffin, you wrap it with plastic, cover it with a towel, and leave it until it is cool. The paraffin baths can be found at medical supply firms.

TENS

Transcutaneous electrical nerve stimulation (TENS) involves the use of electrical stimulation of the nerves to block the pain signals to the brain. It is performed by a professional and is usually done after other methods have been tried and failed. It seems to work best when the pain is in a specific area, such as the lower back. Electrodes are placed on the skin with some gel in the area to be treated. The electrical current is low level and produces a slight, tingling sensation. As with most treatments for pain relief, it does not always work, but it is frequently helpful.

Now let's examine some of the psychological approaches to providing relief for people with arthritis.

Biofeedback

Biofeedback is being taught today by physicians, psychiatrists, psychologists, and many types of therapists. You learn several types of relaxation techniques and by attaching sensitive monitors to your body you can see immediately how your body is reacting to your efforts to relax, lower your blood pressure, diminish your pulse rate, change your temperature, or relax your muscles. Biofeedback reinforces your efforts to control your involuntary reflexes. The monitors let you know if your attempts to "tell your body" what to do are working. Eventually people are able to control these bodily processes without the use of the machine. In Raynaud's phenomenon, for example, you may be able to increase blood flow to your hands or feet. By reducing stress and relaxing tight muscles you may reduce the level of pain and the need for medications.

Deep Breathing

Deep breathing is an effective way to relax. Try to find a time when you will not be disturbed. Find a comfortable, quiet place with as few distractions as possible. Lie down, letting your body be as limp as possible, and close your eyes. Begin breathing very deeply, slowly and rhythmically. Clear your mind of all your problems and distractions. You can concentrate on a word, any word that will help you relax. I personally like to imagine that I am inhaling all the positive energy around me, and when I exhale I am letting go of all the negative things in my life. Inhale, positive, exhale, negative. Try it for 5 or 10 minutes at first and work up to 20 or 30 minutes. You will be amazed how fast the time goes by and how refreshing this method can be.

Positive imagery is another variation of deep breathing. The basic idea is to put yourself in a quiet place with minimal disturbances, close your eyes, relax, and breathe deeply several times. Then imagine that you are in a place where you are happy and relaxed; it might be the beach, the mountains, a cabin in a storm, a boat in calm waters, or whatever place makes you happy. In your mind look carefully at the entire scene. Imagine the smells, the temperature, the sounds, anything you can observe about this happy place. It might mean going back in time to a point in your life when you felt safe and happy. Positive imagery helps you to relax, subdue tensions, and lessen pain.

Self-hypnosis

Again, self-hypnosis is a variation on the above themes. You may need to be taught this technique by a therapist. It is a way to put yourself into a state of deep relaxation. There are audiotapes available in most bookstores to help you with most of these types of deep relaxation. After you have practiced them for a while you will not need the tape. Having practiced these types of techniques, I can actually fall asleep in a chair waiting for my dentist. And believe me, that used to be a very stress-filled time!

A Commonsense Approach

While you need to look very critically at any unproven method of treating arthritis, you might also remember that many of the methods used to treat patients today were once unproven. Not too long ago people with arthritis were sent to bed, whereas today patients are encouraged to be as active as possible. When you have tried just about everything else and you are still in pain and unable to function normally, you may understandably be looking for other possibilities. You need to pay attention to the messages your body sends you. If you are considering an alternative method of treatment, seek the advice of your doctor and see if there is any basis in science for it to work. (If your physician refuses to discuss it, remind him that science doesn't totally understand why aspirin, as well as many other drugs, work.) And above all, be *critical* and be *careful!*

Part Three

TAKING CARE

OF

YOURSELF

The first two parts of the book covered your illness and what you can do about it medically. Now we will introduce you to what you should do for yourself.

12

The Misuse, Overuse, and Underuse Causes of Arthritis

Holding a comb tightly in her left hand as she expertly manipulated my hair, clipping and snipping the ends, Helen Sanchez suddenly winced and lowered her arm. She bent her left thumb and rubbed it gingerly. I saw that the base of her thumb was enlarged and knew she was in pain. I asked her what had happened to her thumb. "Twenty-five years of barbering," she replied, bending her thumb to show its squared-off look.

What Helen showed to me was a left thumb injured during 25 years of misuse by holding her comb too tightly. In addition, she was forced to hold her left arm over her head to position the comb because she was too short for the chair. As we talked more, she told me of the back pain she experienced when she stood too long in that awkward position to hold the comb.

Many work-related injuries like Helen's are similar, regardless of the profession. Dr. Alice Brandfonbrener, a well-known doctor who treats performing arts injuries in Chicago, is an expert on the effects of arthritis on a variety of professionals from cello players to barbers. When I discussed this book with her, she pointed out that people like Helen need to stand in less strained positions and compensate for their misuse. Helen, for example, should build a platform to raise herself off the floor, and she should use the comb underhanded instead of overhand. To reduce the tension on her left thumb and fingers, she can create a customized grip for the comb using a customized grip like Dyna-Form-It putty (see chapter 16) to make the comb easier to hold. She also needs a good exercise program for her back.

It is impossible to estimate how many people have short- and long-term injury to muscles, joints, and all of the other soft tissues such as tendons and ligaments due to improper use or injury. More often than not, a localized pain in a muscle or joint is due to improper use of some kind. One common scenario is the weekend athlete, often a middle-aged man or woman, still remembering past athletic prowess, who tries to play touch football at an office picnic. Another good example is the experience of a friend, Jo Claire Gissel, who was late for her session with her exercise trainer and didn't warm up or stretch her muscles on the stationary bike, treadmill, or Stairmaster. A few days later her knee was so sore that she had to see an orthopedist.

Another scenario is the person who overuses the muscle. Dr. Brandfonbrener helps performing artists when they develop pain in tendons, muscles, or joints that interferes with their performance. For example, if a drummer has pain in his hands, you might say, "Well, he's beating the thing too hard," but the solution is not that simple. Dr. Brandfonbrener looks into the number of repetitions, the intensity of impact on the arms and hands, how the instrument is held, and such things as the physical qualities of the drums' surfaces and the artist's technique. Problems for drummers include tendinitis, nerve entrapments in the wrists, callus problems, and even stress fractures. Hypermobility, or joint laxity, as we discussed in chapter 2, is also a risk factor.

How Misuse, Overuse, and Underuse Affect the Body

When tenderness or pain on motion occurs in muscles, joints, or tendons on a continuing basis, you must become a detective to ferret out the offending activity causing it. Let's look at a few of the major ways that people misuse, overuse, and underuse different parts of the body.

Hands, Fingers, and Wrists

Daily use of a computer for hours on end is a good example of overuse. In writing this book, I experienced this very problem, called *carpal tunnel syndrome*. The first thing I did wrong was to type for an hour or two before the muscles and joints of my hand were ready, thereby triggering muscle spasm in my fingers and wrists. Many people who use computers frequently have inflammation of the wrist and nerve entrapment due to swelling of the wrist. If this is your situation, you need some kind of pad to rest your wrists. The Macintosh computer, for example, has a new PowerBook keyboard with a built-in for the wrist below the keyboard that is part of a handy trackball that replaces the mouse. You hold your wrists in a neutral position with the fingers poised over the keys. It also helps to have a chair you can adjust in height with padded arms. Such features allow you to change your position periodically to reduce fatigue and injury to the wrists and fingers.

Another large group of people who misuse and overuse their fingers, hands, and wrists are assembly-line workers doing repetitive activities such as sewing, inserting, joining, lengthening, bending, winding, or twisting parts or materials. This is an important problem in many jobs, but it can also happen to hobbyists. If you're in this boat, be sure that you don't overuse your fingers and hands. Build up strength in your muscles through exercise to reduce injury.

In short, misuse and overuse have to be a first consideration with any sudden, unexplained pain or swelling of fingers. For example, painting the ceiling for hours with a brush should be number one on your list if you are looking for a cause behind the pain in the fingers and wrist as well as your neck the next day. Piano players and guitarists frequently have trouble with nerve entrapment caused by swelling within the carpal tunnel of the front of the wrist, where nerves to the hand go through.

Elbows

Tennis elbow is a term used by tennis players to describe pain anywhere in the general area of the elbow. The pain begins as you start hitting the ball and can last for days afterward. The usual experience is that the force of the ball being hit transmits up the racket through the hand, wrist, and forearm to the outside of the elbow, creating local injury to the soft tissues around the joint rotary area of the outside edge of the elbow. This is misuse at its worst and is almost always preventable.

Dr. Tom Thornhill, an orthopedist from Boston, feels that there are three main areas of tennis elbow misuse and accompanying injury: the outside, the inside, and the back of the elbow. Each area involves different muscles and the motions of bending and extending the wrist and extending the elbow. There are two ways to power a muscle: *concentric* and *eccentric*. Concentric contraction occurs when the muscle is being shortened, and eccentric contraction occurs when the muscle is being lengthened. The injury to the elbow in tennis elbow is usually due to eccentric contraction, which causes tearing of the tendon and muscle. An example of this is when the forearm is being straightened to hit the ball, and the same forearm muscles while being stretched, are contracted when the ball is hit. Injury occurs as the muscle is being stretched while the muscle fibers are being contracted.

Another way that hitting the tennis ball can injure the elbow is when the fibers of muscle inserting into the bone are pulled away from the bone by too much force from hitting the ball. Injury can be *acute*, which means that it happens suddenly; this kind of initial injury usually gets better on its own after a few weeks. Injury can also be *chronic*, with injury time after time to the muscles, causing shortening of the muscles due to scarring from repeated injury. The usual situation is is *acute/chronic* with recurring episodes of elbow pain lasting for weeks or months. The reason for the flares is that the elbow never gets completely well and is subject to reinjury.

If your pain is in the muscle of the outside of the fleshy part of your forearm, you probably have injured the belly of the muscle during eccentric power contraction; that is, you were stretching the muscle of the forearm when you hit the ball, causing injury. If your pain is where the muscles insert into the bone of the elbow either on the sides or the back, you probably have pulled fibers of tendon from the bone.

Treatment usually includes NSAIDs to reduce pain, and local pressure splints and bandages applied firmly just below the painful area to reduce vibration on the joint and tissues and to absorb the force of the ball as it is being hit. Injection in the elbow with steroids is at times helpful but not as successful as injections in the shoulder.

The best treatment is to figure out what you are doing wrong and correct it. Laying off tennis until the pain disappears allows the body to heal itself; however, the better treatment is to find out what's causing the pain. Start with your racket. Dr. Thornhill and a colleague studied the causes of tennis elbow a few years ago. Of the many possibilities, they were surprised to find that changing tennis rackets was the most frequent event associated with the beginning of tennis elbow. Many players develop tennis elbow by playing with a stiffer racket that does not give when the ball is hit, thereby causing too much transmitted force on your elbow. It is worthwhile therefore to try out a racket first before buying it to be sure that it is safe for you. If a friend has a racket that is the same or similar to the one you're interested in, borrow it and use it for a while. Alternatively, lessen the tension by loosening the strings of the racket. Check your strings to see if they need changing. For club players, gut strings lose their performance in as short a time as a month, so using synthetic strings makes more sense.

If you know that the racket or stringing is not to blame, the cause is likely to be related to your technique of hitting the ball. A common fault is not bending the elbow when hitting the ball to reduce the transmitted force hitting the elbow. If you wait to hit the ball when it is at your side, even with your body, the transmitted force hits more directly on the elbow. The ideal place to hit the ball is when it is just in front of your body, causing you to lean forward, but if you hit it when it is too far in front of you, your elbow will be too straight because you are swinging too far out. Also, by hitting the ball when it is close to the front of your body, you are using the forward force of your entire body and not overusing your forearm. There are many ways that your technique of hitting the ball can be wrong, and a good tennis teacher can solve them in a hurry.

A major way to prevent tennis elbow is to stretch your arm muscles properly before playing. Extend your elbow, pronate (turn your hand over with the palm down), and fully flex your wrist, bending your fingers toward the palm. Hold for a count of 5, and repeat several times. Remember to stretch those leg muscles too.

Another major way to prevent problems is to build up strength in the arm muscles. Most health clubs have a Cybex, which is a bar that you can roll forward by flexing the wrists and roll backward by extending the wrists using a 2-pound weight. There is also a handle for you to pronate and supinate (turn the hand over and up again). You can do approximately the same by wringing a wet hand towel one way and then the other. In the next chapter on exercise we'll discuss this in more detail. To reassure you in your quest to control tennis elbow, Dr. Thornhill feels that only 2 percent of people with chronic tennis elbow ever need surgery.

Misuse and overuse of the elbow is not limited to tennis players, as tennis elbow or its equivalent is also present in golf enthusiasts and even in Little League baseball players. If you have children in the Little League age group, you should be aware that overuse pitching by young boys or girls can injure the elbow. The Little League has rules about the number of pitches that can be made in a game by pitchers of certain age groups, so if you have a pitcher in your house, be aware.

Shoulders

Dr. Thornhill points out that the majority of nontraumatic conditions afflicting the shoulder are caused by tendinitis in the cuff or sleeve that holds the shoulder together. In people in their twenties, overuse of the arm with overhead motion such as throwing balls or hitting balls with a tennis racket causes local bleeding and swelling of the shoulder cuff due to rubbing of tendons on bone. Another name for this is *tendinitis impingement syndrome,* or "pitcher's arm." If the overuse and misuse continue, scarring and inflammation of the tendons can occur in later years. After many years of continued overuse, the tendons may rupture, and scarring will cause loss of motion unless surgery is performed. The best treatment is to stop irritating the shoulder with overuse. Although NSAIDs can help the pain and steroid injections can reduce inflammation and pain, rest and discontinuation of the misuse are essential.

Another frequent afflication of the shoulder happens to be my problem. My left shoulder area has always been so much lower than the right that tailors altering suits always have to pad the shoulders. In Houston, my exercise trainer, David Taylor, gave me an exercise with weights to increase the size of the trapezius muscle that slopes from the neck to the shoulder. While discussing this section of the book with Dr. Thornhill, I mentioned my shoulder problem, which has been present since my early teen years. He quickly figured out what I had done wrong to misuse my shoulder. Growing up, I delivered newspapers to homes twice daily for several years. I carried a heavy bag of papers slung over my right shoulder and threw the papers onto the porches of houses from the sidewalk. I threw a lot of papers during those years. What happened to me is called *drooping shoulder* caused by a laxity of the capsule of the shoulder joint due to repeated stretching from throwing papers in my situation. When the doctor pulled down on my left upper arm, I felt it pull out of the socket. This condition is very common among tennis players, pitchers, and anyone doing repetitive motions of the shoulder. The treatment, of course, is prevention.

Hips, Knees, Legs, and Feet

The main overuse and misuse occurring in these areas involve a great American pastime: running and jogging. As we pointed out earlier, a force of four to eight times your body weight is exerted on the hips, knees, and legs during jumping or running. This fact of physics means that you must have proper warm-up periods, stretching, conditioning of the body, and use of proper shoes.

Runner's knee is a specific problem for runners. The lump of bone located just below your kneecap, called the tibial tuberosity, is subject to local stress and trauma with pain and swelling. Shin splints are a variation of the same injury to the covering of the bone over the shins. Running on a hard concrete surface such as a paved street is often the cause. *Achilles tendinitis* is inflammation of the heel cord and is more serious than the bone-covering problems just described because the heel cord may actually rupture while running. A bad sign is if your knees swell with fluid every time you jog. Stress fractures in the feet are also common disorders for dedicated runners. The strong plantar fascia and ligament running the length of the sole of the foot can be traumatized and become inflamed due to poorly fitting shoes or foot abnormalities.

Prevention is the main treatment for all these problems. First, you must have properly fitting shoes and socks; tennis shoes are not OK. Be sure that you get help from a qualified person for the right type of running shoes *for you*. Second, be sure to condition, stretch, and warm up to prevent stress injuries to the legs and joints. If you try to run full speed on cold muscles and tendons, you'll pay for it with pain or injury. If you do develop swelling of the knees with fluid or pain in the legs every time you run, your body is telling you something. Please take up the identical exercise in a swimming pool and save those joints. The effect on your health and conditioning is the same.

The Back

The back is often subject to underuse with resulting muscular weakness and low back pain. Statistics vary, but low back pain with no demonstrable cause is at least one of the most common afflictions. In a family practice study of patients over a three-year period, 10 percent of men and women had sufficiently painful low back pain to bring them to the doctor. Some reports say that up to 80 percent of people have low back pain at some time in their lives. Many orthopedists tell me that low back pain is the single most frequent complaint encountered in their practices.

It is impressive to see how many people can lose their low back pain with no apparent cause when they are persuaded to follow a strengthening program for their backs on a regular basis. Strengthening the back muscles does reduce, if not eliminate, low back pain more often than not. My favorite exercise for this is the Roman chair used in health clubs. This is a frame at about a 45-degree angle that supports your body from the feet to the groin area. You bend over to the floor and up, usually starting with eight repetitions, then stopping, counting to five, and repeating two times. As you grow stronger, you increase repetitions. If you feel pain, you reduce by one repetition until no pain is produced. Using this exercise on a daily basis, your back pain has the best chance to disappear as the muscles become stronger to hold the back. By building up the endurance and strength of the back muscles, you can delay or eliminate the pain of fatigue.

Other ways to achieve strengthening include abdominal exercises and stretching exercises. The next chapter, devoted to exercise, will provide more details.

13

Staying Fit and Energized

Movement and Exercise for Everyone

In an article in *Arthritis Today,* Maxine Rock, the award-winning author of four books, shared with all of us the big change she underwent 15 years ago with her spinal arthritis. Her medicines weren't helping, her stiffness was crippling her activities, and life was not getting better. She summoned her courage, slipped on her running shoes, and began running two miles three times a week. Much to her wonder, the omnipresent pain and stiffness in her back and neck almost disappeared in a few months. What is surprising about Maxine's experience is that when she began her exercise program of running, people with ankylosing spondylitis were being told to take it easy and save those joints. We know now, of course, that exercise is not only helpful, but it also may be the best thing you'll ever do to help your arthritis.

Some Basics About Exercise

Exercise gives power to your muscles, endurance to your body, and flexibility to your joints. The result includes feeling better every day, reducing pain in your joints, and lifting your spirits. Not only is the pain reduced, but you feel better and become stronger with more stamina.

Fortunately, there are many ways to exercise. You do not have to jog or run to make your life fuller, happier, and more productive. As you read the following ideas, take note of the many options available to you. Remember, *not* embarking on a successful exercise plan for you is not one of your options.

Let's first spend a little time talking about different terms used in the exercise world. *Power* is the same as strength, referring to a muscle or a muscle group, such as the strength shown by a weightlifter when he or she uses his or her arms. Strengthening muscles around joints reduces the strain on the joints and capsules, holding them together, and prevents injury from sudden twists and turns as well as from heavy weight-bearing.

There are two main exercises to build power in your muscles: isometric and isotonic. When you do isometric exercises, you tighten your muscles but don't move or strain your joints. Examples are squeezing or tightening your leg muscles or creating resistance by pressing one palm against the other. Isotonic exercises involve moving your joint as you tighten the muscle, such as straightening your knee while sitting in a chair. Resistance isotonic exercise involves application of an opposite force, or resistance, to straightening the knee or elbow. This can be done by pushing against the extending knee or, more accurately, by using equipment that creates and measures resistance. The equipment found at health clubs allows you to progressively increase your strength under supervision of qualified trainers.

Endurance of muscles relates to the fitness of not only the muscles but also the stamina of your body. In addition to the special muscle fibers that control strength, side by side in the same muscle, there are special muscle fibers of the body that govern endurance. Exercises that improve endurance and general fitness of the body are called *aerobic*, and include running, walking, and swimming. The term *aerobic* is used because long-term muscular endurance needs oxygen from the blood to replenish oxygen used in exercise, so improving oxygen consumption by the body is the way to increase endurance or stamina. *Anaerobic*, or quick and sudden muscular movement, uses stored energy in the muscle and is therefore limited in duration of action and is the mechanism of power exercise.

Flexibility of joints is essential for normal motion and is the key issue in exercise programs directed toward maintaining and improving your joint motion. For instance, did you notice several runners dropping out of their races with muscular pain during the 1992 summer Olympics? Some of them probably had failed to warm up properly. Warming up includes stretching your muscles and tendons by doing flexibility exercises or joint range-of-motion exercises. Following the warm-up period, the maximum heavy exercise time for increasing power or endurance begins. However, before stopping, slow down the pace of exercise for a cool-down period of several minutes to prevent stiffness or pain of muscles later.

General Fitness Exercises

To give you a sense of where we are heading in our discussion of exercise, let me give you an overview of a program that I feel is essential for you to incorporate into your life. No matter how limited you may be right now, everything we'll discuss about general fitness applies to you, although you need to tailor it to what you can do now.

The single most important activity is working on *posture*. We'll cover some of the more important *endurance exercises* such as walking, jogging, swimming, bicycling, and stair climbing. Next will be *power exercises* including resistance equipment used at health clubs to increase your muscular strength. Finally, we'll help you design your own program by detailing the daily exercise program that works for me, a 64-year-old, over-the-hill rheumatologist who has more aches, pains, and stiffness than he cares to admit.

Posture

There is nothing more important than good posture to prevent many aches and pains resulting from improper pressure on joints and muscles. Posture goes beyond the oft-heard command to "suck in your gut, roll those shoulders back, tuck in your fanny, and let's see that head and neck stiff and straight." At the beginning of the chapter, I mentioned *Arthritis Today*, an excellent magazine written and published by the Arthritis Foundation, that you should read for ideas (see Appendix 1). An article on posture by Tracy Ballew, who interviewed a physical therapist, Victoria Gall of Boston, is the most practical and succinct that I've seen in a long time, and I'm going to share their ideas with you, adding a few ideas of my own.

Standing. Stand in front of a full-length mirror, and look at yourself from front and side. Do the following:
- Distribute your weight equally on both feet.
- Point your feet forward or slightly outward.
- Straighten your knees, leaving a little space between them. Don't lock them.

- Roll your shoulders back so that they are level and relaxed.
- Tuck that tummy in.
- Run an imaginary string down your head, neck, and spine.
  Use it to keep your body straight.

Walking. To insure the proper posture for gait, look at yourself in a mirror while you are walking. A few points make all of the difference in the world:

- Take steps of equal length.
- Make sure that you have a heel–to–toe gait,
  and that you bend your knees.
- Swing your arms naturally by your sides.
- Make sure that your shoes fit properly, are comfortable,
  and provide good support. A good shoe salesperson
  can tell you if it's a good fit, but only you can tell if
  it's comfortable.

Sitting. In the previous chapter, we discussed the effects of computers and proper sitting. Sitting is important. Your chair must fit you, meaning that your feet must touch the floor. The chair ideally should be adjustable in height so that your arms are not strained when typing. Arm rests are helpful in reducing fatigue. Sit up straight when working in a chair, and be sure that your back is properly supported and rested. Slumping makes you tire faster. If I sit improperly at the computer, my upper back muscles start to hurt because of spasm.

Another problem not generally mentioned with sitting properly is using glasses. I need to wear bifocals, and when I typed at the computer, my neck arched in extension to compensate for looking over the lower part of my glasses; it caused a lot of muscular neck pain. I solved it by having a pair of glasses made for computer use only that are set for 22 inches focal point and are not bifocal. (The usual reading glasses are set for 14 inches focal point, but the additional 8 inches compensate for being farther from the screen because of the keyboard.) The computer-reading glasses eliminated my neck muscle fatigue immediately.

Lying down. Victoria Gall recommends that you should fall asleep in a position that is comfortable for you, noting that you should not end up in a twisted, awkward position that strains your muscles. For years I always had a pain here or there from falling asleep in a twisted position. You can change that most habitual position, however. I did. Just experiment with different positions. Most people can fall asleep in a curled-up position. The standard recommendation is to have a firm mattress. To me, the goal is to wake up refreshed and rejuvenated, and if a soft mattress or a waterbed makes the difference, use it.

Endurance Exercises

Endurance exercise increases stamina by improving oxygen consumption by the body and in particular improving oxygen consumption of the muscles. We know that planned endurance exercise does improve stamina. We also know that even people in their seventies and eighties can increase body muscle mass and decrease body fat mass with regular endurance exercise. The vast majority of people in this age group ought to be active and look great.

No matter what your age, you need to be participating in general fitness on a regular basis. All of the endurance exercises we discuss here are useful, and all can be used in your program to reduce boredom.

Walking and jogging. Walking is the least strenuous of the endurance exercises, but you should not diminish its importance. Walking one to three miles three times weekly, a minimal commitment to health, will help you feel and look better and add years to your life. You can walk even if you need a cane or walker. Just adapt the exercise to what you can do and for how long you can do it. (Refer to chapter 16 for information on walking canes.) There are many advantages to walking that make it practical for most people. It's certainly easier on your joints than jogging. It requires no special skills or expensive equipment. No matter where you are, you can find a place to walk. For years my wife and I walked around the Galleria shopping mall in Houston on Sunday mornings in the winter, which not only protected us from the rainy, cold weather but also allowed us to look at the hundreds of store windows during our three-mile hike. Even if you use a cane, walker, or crutches, walking can be a great fitness exercise.

However, give yourself a chance to build up to how far and how long you can walk or jog. Start slowly with regard to time and distance, and build up your endurance. This means starting with 10-minute walks on level paths. If you're out of breath after this, start with 5 minutes. Remember: the amount of time that you walk needs to be increased to 30 to 45 minutes as a goal. After reaching 30 to 45 minutes' duration, pick up the pace and walk faster until you can do three miles in 45 minutes. That's plenty fast and long enough to get the job done. Added features are to pick walking places that are uphill and downhill to increase your endurance training.

One special problem that you may need to address is what kind of shoe to wear. The easiest thing to do is to check out the many walking shoes made by such companies as Reebok or Nike to find the proper fit for you, following the advice of the shoe person. Be sure they are comfortable when you buy them; shoes that aren't comfortable when you buy them often stay that way. If you have cramps in your legs or painful knees after walking, pull back on either the time or pace of walking; you may need to warm up before walking, walk more slowly, or stretch your legs by doing squats—bending at the ankles and knees—a few times before starting.

Another way to walk or run which allows you to measure and control your speed and distance is to use the treadmill equipment at a health club. The treadmill has programs that control not only how many miles per hour you walk, but also what degree of steepness you climb. Some machines offer planned programs that vary speed and steepness and include warm-up and cool-down periods. You can use this program to your advantage to gradually build up your endurance, which is what I do. If you could see the many men and women in their sixties, seventies, and even eighties with arthritis using the treadmill at the University Club in Houston, you would realize that exercise is not something limited to younger people.

Swimming and other water exercises. If you are in the unfortunate situation of having a great deal of restricted joint motion or you have too much pain to walk, much less participate in a power exercise program, then here is where you start your exercise path to a better life with more endurance and better joint motion. Because of its buoyancy, water exercise helps the pain go away because gravity is not relentlessly pressing on the joints. You feel free for the first time in years, and because of reduced or absent pain, you feel OK about moving all of your joints. If you are like a fish and grew up swimming laps, have at it; you'll be way ahead of the game. If you otherwise need a blueprint showing you how to take advantage of water to improve your fitness, reduce your pain, and improve motion in those joints that are restricted, hire an instructor. Remember to do at least 20 minutes of laps three or four times a week (or more if you can).

Many arthritis sufferers feel a little uneasy in the water, and people who have limited motion and joint pain on land sometimes worry about drowning. However, the AquaJogger is really helpful, especially if you use it regularly and consistently. (See page 33 for details and ordering information.)

On your first day, aquajog only a few minutes in the deep water, then increase the time daily. With this device, remember that it is unnecessary to walk on the bottom. Using the Aqua-Jogger is a sensible way to increase your strength and endurance. The flotation device, made of a synthetic foam, does not absorb water and fits around your middle back. It is attached to an elastic belt that fits snugly around the tummy. It is reminiscent of the old ski belts used many years ago. It was developed in the 1980s for competitive runners and other athletes to speed recovery from injuries to arms and legs. The exercises are the same as on land but have the advantage of the buoyancy of water to eliminate the painful injury inflicted by gravity on land. You can see that your needs are the same as the world-class runners with respect to your joints.

There are several basic water exercises to try: running and walking, upper body exercises, cross-country skiing, and leg raises. The body alignment for running and walking is the same as for land—upright with a slight forward lean. Move your arms and legs the same as on land. The upper body exercises consist of cupping your hands with the palms facing forward and backward as you move your arms in different directions. In doing the cross-country skiing exercise, the legs and arms are extended and straight with a scissoring motion of your legs from the hips and another scissoring motion from the shoulders for the arms. In the leg raises, you lie on your back. Position your body at a 45-degree angle, using your arms for balance as you bring your legs to your chest. The AquaJogger instructional brochure gives training tips that are both useful and sensible. Here are a few:

- Begin sessions with a *warm-up* consisting of easy, smooth, flowing motions for 10 minutes or more.
- The *main session* can consist of continuous aerobic activity where you maintain an exertion level that allows you to keep

your breathing under control, or a series of exercises with short intervals of rest in between, or specific exercises followed by intervals of rest. Always work within your established medical limits with the objective of working up to at least 20 minutes of quality training.

- The main session is followed by a *cool-down* of 7 to 10 minutes of easy, fluid movements in the water followed by some static (fixed, at rest) stretches, emphasizing those muscle groups employed during the session.
- Pay particular attention to your body alignment and keep your body in a proper workout position.
- As you become comfortable with the exercises, work more powerfully against the water's resistance.
- Increase intensity by using as much of the water's surface as possible and by using larger motions. Do this gradually with special attention to any strain on joints caused by the increased resistance.
- When in doubt, be conservative. Stay behind the point of pain and just "nudge" the level of intensity each day. A sudden increase can result in injury.
- Always consult your physician in establishing your personal guidelines and limitations.

Keep these alternatives in mind as well: The AquaJogger can be reversed and the large area worn on the front with the buckle in the back. This works well for when you are swimming on your stomach or snorkeling. You can also change the focus of the flotation by turning the AquaJogger upside down with the foam hump pointed down rather than up the back. This position is sometimes used by children or short people who have a small back areas.

Other water exercises that save wear and tear on your joints include water aerobics classes as well as lap swimming. As stated at the beginning, if you have significant problems with your joints, the easiest and best way to get started with your exercise program is in the water.

Bicycling. Stationary bicycling or riding a real bike offers an attractive alternative to jogging, walking, or swimming. If your joint problems are minor and you are reasonably flexible in motion, riding a bicycle on the street is certainly more fun because you can enjoy the fresh air and scenery. It is most important that you observe the same rules as in walking and water exercise; that is, you should warm up at the beginning and cool down at the end. If you are older, concerns about falling and breaking a hip or arm may make bicycling unattractive to you.

Riding the right bicycle is important. The pedals must allow each leg to be straight, with the ball of your foot resting on the pedal at the bottom position. The seat must be comfortable. Your arms should be comfortably bent at the elbow when you are holding the handlebar grips. Your back should be relaxed and comfortable. There are many other things you will need to know about bicycling in today's world. Bicycles have become so individualized that you will benefit by visiting a bicycle store and acquainting yourself with gears, dropped handlebars, all-terrain or mountain bikes, and special seats for the squeamish. If you see that biking on the streets and paths is for you, remember that the rules for endurance exercise are the same.

Stationary bicycles are more user-friendly and come either upright or horizontal. They're not so expensive that home use is impossible. You can read, watch the news or soaps on TV, or rent a movie. They are an attractive alternative to a health club. Remember to measure for the proper height of the seat so that your legs are straight when you are at the bottom of the pedaling cycle. Also remember that you must warm up before and cool down at the end. Twenty to 30 minutes is enough.

Stair climbing. No one in our circle of acquaintances who is not in training for the decathlon or an NFL football team does stair climbing in the bleachers. In fact, stair climbing may be the ultimate exercise both for endurance and power of the legs. The place where stair climbing comes into its own is at a health club using mechanical stair-climbing equipment. Several different types of machines are geared to climb as many stairs as quickly as you want, for as long as you want, and in different sequences. This is mainly an aerobic exercise but does contribute to strength of muscles. Start slowly and build up from 5 minutes to 20 minutes. When you've arrived at a 20-minute time, add resistance to the climb. Never add time and resistance on the same day. We'll talk more about how you do this later. Suffice it to say that you need an exercise trainer to plan stair climbing for you, at least initially.

Power Exercises

A planned program to increase the strength of your muscles is essential to feeling better, having less pain, and increasing joint strength and flexibility. Isometric, or squeezing exercises, are good for maintenance of strength, but isotonic exercises (exercises that push against resistance) will give the most results in the least amount of time. When you've achieved your goal of increased strength, then maintenance power exercise is necessary two or three times weekly.

Resistance can take the form of simply pushing one hand against the other or using your body weight as a resistive force of gravity. You can use the Roman chair back-strengthening exercise where you lean your upper body over a padded table angled at 45 degrees, touch the floor, and then extend the back. Another form of isotonic exercise is the use of weights or dumbbells. These are particularly useful in building strength in the upper back and arms.

The most important power exercise system to me is the Cybex

or Nautilus equipment that allows a progressive, graded, and systematic approach to getting stronger. The equipment looks a little scary and formidable, but it is actually simple to use. The Cybex and Nautilus people simply added known weight-opposing resistance to many of the standard stretching and flexibility exercises that you and I knew about from grade school onward. These exercises include knee extension, rowing, leg and arm curls, sit-ups, arm extension, neck stretching, wrist motion in all directions, weight lifting, squeezing the elbows together and then the shoulder blades, pelvic tilts, back lifts, and various stretching exercises for the legs.

To obtain the most benefit from power exercise, the game plan to follow is to sign up with a health club and a trainer, which is usually included with your first few visits. She or he will assess your exercise goals, and then the two of you will plan a program of progressive strengthening exercises. Usually this will involve teaching you how to use the endurance equipment and the power-strengthening exercise equipment. You will probably use about 10 pieces of equipment per session. For example, if you use the leg extension exercise, you might start with a certain weight of 4 pounds of resistance. While seated, you push against the bar to extend your legs. The bar has the known 4 pounds of weight resistance to your extension. You will do the exercise for 8 repetitions, pause for a count of 5, and then repeat two more times with a pause in between. You only do the strengthening exercises every other day to give the muscles a chance to rest. When you have done the exercise on three occasions, you increase the number of repetitions to 10 and then to 12 after three more occasions. There is nothing to be gained by doing more than 12 repetitions of any exercise. At 12 repetitions, add a half pound or 1 pound of weight to the system. Never increase repetitions and add weight at the same time.

If you feel pain the day after you exercise, your muscles are telling you that you've done too much. Pull back what you are doing to the previous level. It is important not to attempt exercise with equipment unless a qualified trainer trains you in the proper use of the equipment.

A Sample Exercise Program

The information presented in this chapter may be a little over-whelming in that many options are open to you in your quest for better health through exercise. What is best for me probably is not best for you, but a run-through of my personal program may help you to organize your own plan for exercise. Remember, I am 64 years old and not athletic. Also, it is important for you to visit several health clubs to see if you like the atmosphere and are comfortable with the clients and the trainers. Some clubs cater more to older people and some to younger; however, most are interested in all ages.

My weekly exercise program was recently updated by David Taylor, an exercise trainer at the University Club in Houston. David has been extremely helpful to me in my drive toward better physical fitness. I try to work out every morning Monday through Friday. On Mondays, Wednesdays, and Fridays I do endurance exercise. I try to limit my time to 30 to 40 minutes. I alternate between the Stairmaster, arm exerciser (upper extremity ergometer), bicycle, treadmill, and AquaJogger. On Mondays and Fridays I do one of the equipment exercises for 20 minutes and another for 5 minutes. I finish with stretching and strengthening exercises: the Roman chair for stretching and strengthening the back, abdominal exercises, and stretching exercises of the legs and arms. On Wednesdays I aquajog in the pool for 30 minutes, always remembering to warm up and cool down each time.

On Tuesdays and Thursdays I work on my power exercise plan. David outlined for me how much weight resistance and how many repetitions for each exercise. He also outlined how to increase both the weights and repetitions in the same manner. The equipment I use includes the leg press, where I push against a weighted resistance and straighten my legs; the rowing machine; the leg curl, where I bend my legs while lying down against weights; the lateral pull-down of an overhead weight for back exercise; the Roman chair described earlier for back stretch and strengthening; 8-pound weights I lift for arm strength; the triceps curl and triceps extension; the leg extension while seated against weight; the shoulder press; abdominal exercises; stretching exercises; and finally, 6-pound weights lifted in a special position for my left trapezius back muscle (I have a drooping left shoulder).

This varied program does not become dull, and each part contributes to my general fitness. If I develop muscular or joint pain after a session, I cut back on the exercise that seems to be the culprit. If I can't figure it out, I ask David. The biggest obstacle to success is not having the perseverance to keep it up. The reason that I do continue is that I feel better each day when I do the exercises. Another reason for me is that if I lay off for a week, my back begins to hurt again when I try to sleep at night.

By the way, before you use them, let me address a few of the usual excuses when it comes to exercise:

Excuse: It's dull.
Remedy: Change the routine frequently.

Excuse: My arthritis is giving me fits today.
Remedy: Cut back on your exercise. Don't skip it.

Excuse: It takes too much time.
Remedy: Nonsense. All of us make time for what's important.

Excuse: It hurts.
Remedy: Cut back on your routine.

Excuse: I don't see any results.
Remedy: Use a progressive plan to gain strength and endurance, and you will see results weekly.

Note: I firmly believe that specific exercises to correct deformities of joints or muscles should be planned by your rheumatologist, orthopedist, rehab doctor, or physical therapist. The general fitness program outlined above will prevent many deformities and improve strength and motion, but if you have special exercises for a knee or wrist, do those; however, don't let up on your general fitness program.

Yoga

Most western minds think of yoga as something you do in a turban and loincloth, with a body contorted into unreal, impossible shapes. Yoga exercises are not usually that extreme when practiced in this country. Kathy's experience with yoga (she took classes when she was pregnant with her second child) is that it is a terrific way to gently stretch muscles and increase flexibility, and at the same time it provides a sense of enervation, tranquility, and inner peace. It incorporates a type of meditation, or focusing on the inner self, to achieve serenity and well-being.

Many of the health clubs now offer classes in yoga, primarily teaching the different yoga postures (asanas) and the breathing exercises (pranayamas). There are also many individuals who teach the different types of yoga exercises. Yoga is a good part of an overall program of fitness. While it is not aerobic, it will certainly prepare you for other exercises by stretching your muscles and loosening your body.

T'ai Chi Ch'uan

Kathy highly recommends this ancient Chinese practice for people with arthritis. There have been pictures of multitudes of Chinese people, including the very young and the very old, doing these rhythmic, graceful movements. This type of exercise is especially popular in California. The first time Kathy saw someone performing the motions was on a beach in Big Sur, but she has also seen people on beaches in Chicago performing these movements.

T'ai chi ch'uan is described as "body and mind in harmony." It has been practiced in China for almost a thousand years. It is a type of moving meditation related to the Chinese philosophy of maintaining a healthy body and a healthy mind in harmony with nature. It is becoming increasingly popular in this country and it is fairly easy to find instructors to teach you.

Whichever type of exercise you choose, develop a program and follow it diligently. If there is one thing we know about arthritis, it's that *exercise helps!*

14

Arthritis Cuisine

Chances are that you're as confused as we are about what scientists and doctors recommend we should and should not eat. In fact, if you were to review articles from recent books, magazines, and newspapers, you could justify almost any diet or food that exists.

For most of my life I have been one of those people for whom food was important, especially the taste: I was sick to learn that fried eggs, buttered white toast, and salty, peppered bacon full of fat were no-no's. And to top it off, my wife started serving Basic 4 cereal with bananas at breakfast. (I have to attend my men's breakfast club each week to get eggs Benedict and French toast dripping with butter and syrup.)

The probability is that you too fall from grace and are not always perfect in following the rules of proper diet. Fortunately, cooler heads prevail, and we are all forced to face up to the fact that proper diet and nutrition not only affect our health and longevity but may reduce the severity of some diseases, including many kinds of arthritis. All it takes is some self-discipline and the knowledge that we can no longer ignore our diets and waistlines if we want to live longer.

In this chapter, we are going to talk about general nutritional concerns, weight control (this is probably the most common, serious, and vexing problem), nutritional diet modification to improve arthritis, and the fascinating story of how vitamins, minerals, and some food allergies may affect your arthritis.

General Nutritional Issues

Most people have had training in the food exchange charts that "simplify" figuring out how much to eat. Some charts indicate that we should eat about 30 percent fat, 20 percent protein, and 50 percent carbohydrate. Unfortunately, labels on foods are often confusing about how much fat, sugar, and protein are present. Few of us carry a calculator or even want to carry one to figure out how much to eat.

After much give-and-take between the Department of Agriculture and the meat industry, new guidelines were recently issued that use a triangular pyramid shape to help people remember the five basic foods and one no-no:

Fats, sugars, and oils (seldom, unless you can't stand it)

Milk, cheese, and yogurt   2 servings/day

Meat, fish, poultry, eggs, and beans   2 servings/day

Vegetables   3 to 5 servings/day

Bread, cereal, rice, and pasta   6 to 11 servings/day

Fruits   2 to 4 servings/day

This chart can help you remember how to eat well. The Department of Agriculture, a host of other organizations, and many national magazines publish detailed food charts with caloric values that you can also use. One problem is that there is no uniformity of opinion regarding how large a serving should be. To give you some idea of how much one serving equals, use this table:

Fruits (strawberries, peaches)	½ cup
Rice or cereal	1 cup
Vegetables (corn, peas, etc.)	½ cup
Fish, meat, or poultry	3 to 4 ounces
Yogurt or milk products	½ cup frozen, 1 cup fresh

These serving counts are probably the easiest to remember; however, if you're counting calories, you can go by these rules:
- 1,600 calories are thought to represent a reasonable amount for sedentary people and some older adults.
- 2,200 calories daily represent a satisfactory amount for active people, including teenagers.
- 2,800 calories daily or more may be necessary for extremely active adults and teenage boys.

To derive the calorie count, first look at the chart or label on the can or box to see how many grams of fat, protein, or carbohydrate are in each serving. You now need to remember that there are 4 calories in each gram of protein or carbohydrate and 9 calories in each gram of fat. Using a calculator, you can figure what the total calorie count is for one portion or serving. For example, if you eat a normal serving of grade A fancy chopped spinach (frozen), the label states that a normal serving is 3.3 ounces, containing 20 calories, 3 grams of protein, 3 grams of carbohydrate, and 0 grams of fat. So 3 grams of protein multiplied by 4 calories equals 12 calories, and 3 grams of carbohydrate multiplied by 4 calories equals 12 calories. One serving equals 24 calories. The box says 20 calories, but that is an estimate.

The only other major rule to live by is *no salt*. There is so much salt in the food we eat. You can substitute any one of hundreds of spices and condiments instead of adding more salt. Watch out for hidden and unsuspected sources of salt in prepared foods such as frozen food and processed canned food. Whenever possible, use fresh vegetables and fruits, as they are much better for you. For example, an ordinary serving of baked potato has 1 milligram of salt while the same amount of potato chips has 1,000 milligrams. Watch out for condiments such as tomato ketchup; they're loaded with salt (much to my dismay).

Many people also don't realize that alcohol is a complex sugar and adds loads of calories! So cut down on before-dinner drinks. Avoid saturated fat as much as possible. Adding plain sugar for sweetening should be limited. Most people use artificial sweeteners such as Equal or Sweet'N Low.

Weight Control

I have to watch my weight, as do many people when they reach a certain age. What I do is to weigh myself on a good scale each morning before breakfast. I try to adhere to the general rules given above with regard to quantity and quality of food, and let my weight guide me to maintain those rules as a way of life instead of waiting until I've added 10 pounds and try to crash diet the problem. One major component of weight control is what we've discussed in detail in the preceding chapter: exercise. Weight is a balance of food intake and exercise output, so decreasing those foods that you know are doing it to you and increasing your energy output are the keys to success.

One compelling reason for you to control weight if you have arthritis of the knees, ankles, or hips is that every extra pound of weight adds four times more stress on the joints when you run, walk, or jump. This weight adds injury to the joint, and so reducing your weight is a major step you can take to make your arthritis better. In addition to reducing the strain on the joints, proper weight lessens pain and generally improves how you feel about yourself.

Unfortunately, there is no magic way to lose weight; it simply requires determination to do the right thing so that you can feel better and look better. Of course, this is easier said than done. We've heard about all the methods, from Pritikin, to Ultra Slim-Fast to Weight Watchers, but the data about all such programs suggest what really works is self-discipline and willpower. That means controlling those impulses to snack and graze in the kitchen.

Begin by reviewing your normal diet and commit to reducing your salt, fat, and carbohydrate intake. When I want to lose a few excess pounds, I stop my evening drink before dinner and my red wine with dinner. While it doesn't sound like much, in four or five days, my weight is back to normal. We all know which foods do it to us, and what quantity is too much.

A big problem for many people is the enormous portions of food served in restaurants. If you need to eat out, consider sharing. It's not embarrassing to be healthy and alive. For years, my wife and I felt embarrassed about ordering only two salads and one entree, but we do that now without hesitation. Another ploy is to order two salads, two appetizers, and no main course. Lastly, stay away from those rich desserts unless you compensate for them with less food earlier in the meal.

Nutritional
Diet Modification

Literally hundreds of foods and combinations of foods have been suggested over the centuries to help the pain and swelling of arthritis. Few stand the test of time. Today the fad is fish oils. Some believe that eicosanoids, components of cold-water fish oil, affect the arachidonic acids in the body that control inflammation and arthritis. Dr. Dwight Robinson of Boston points out that in at least eight well-controlled studies, people with arthritis experienced mild improvement with fish oils, but the results are not very impressive in his view. Also, even though fish oil is a food, its use as an arthritis drug must be approved by the FDA. Since this has not occurred, caution is recommended.

Note especially that cod liver oil is *not* OK to use, because it has too much vitamin A. Oil from cold-water fish seems to be better and has more omega-3 polyunsaturated fatty acids that affect the arachidonic acid cycle in the body. You can purchase preparations in gelatin capsules.

Nutritional modification has proved successful especially in the treatment of gout. People with gout need to reduce or eliminate the glandular meats, such as pancreas (sweetbreads) and, of course, alcohol.

One new diet supplement for people with arthritis being evaluated by Dr. Robert Zurier of Worcester, Massachusetts, is gamma-linolenic acid (GLA). This also is a polyunsaturated fatty acid that may alter the arachidonic acid cycle of inflammation in the body. It is too soon to know how helpful this will be.

Food Allergies That Affect Arthritis

For years doctors have known that selected food antigens can be found in the blood of sensitive people. Occasionally a patient with RA will clearly have serious flares of arthritis when exposed to milk or other foods. These cases are different from highly allergic individuals who get serum sickness—which includes short-lived arthritis—from chemicals such as penicillin or foods such as shell-fish. Dr. Richard Panush of New Jersey, has also conducted several studies of people with RA who thought that they had flares of arthritis after eating different foods, including milk. It was clear that they were right, and several had flares of several days' duration after exposure to the offending food on a recurring basis.

This does not conclusively mean, however, that allergies cause RA. They can trigger a flare but do not cause it or cure it. So don't rush out to try one of the myriad diets that "cure" arthritis by cutting out certain foods. Many diets may help a little bit for a little while, and there are many adherents to the idea that RA is caused by a particular food. Over the years I explored a number of diets and allergy regimens that hoped to cure arthritis by removing one set of foods or another and I found them too often disappointing. Food allergy does not cause destructive, erosive arthritis, so keep eating those foods that you want according to appropriate health and nutritional guidelines.

Vitamins, Minerals, and Trace Elements

There has been a tremendous surge of interest by physicians, research scientists, and people in general in discovering whether minimal deficiencies of vitamins, minerals, and trace elements cause human illness. Unfortunately, we have no major conclusions, but let's review what we know.

Vitamins are chemicals from outside the body that help the body regulate many basic chemical reactions such as converting food into energy. At least 13 such reactions are known. There is no question that they are important to maintain and improve good health. For example, we know that vitamin C, or ascorbic acid, found in fruits and leafy vegetables prevents scurvy because when a marked deficiency occurs, the disease results. For years, Linus Pauling has extolled the intake of large doses of vitamin C to cure colds. As far as vitamin C and RA are concerned, in at least one study vitamin C was deficient in the serum of RAs, and immunoenhancement was reduced in test-tube experiments. However, while the poor immune response was corrected in the test tube by the addition of Vitamin C, the arthritis of RA did not improve with the use of vitamin C in the studies that were done.

Vitamins E and beta-carotene (a precursor of vitamin A), together with vitamin C, are known as *antioxidants* and act as guards to neutralize chemical radicals in the blood that participate in the immune response that affects arthritis. Like vitamin C, it is not known whether these two vitamins help people with RA. Vitamin K helps in the clotting of the blood but also helps to retain calcium in the bone. Vitamin D affects bone formation. None of these, however, has been shown to have any specific, positive effect on arthritis.

Many people also believe that trace minerals such as zinc and copper help reduce the severity of arthritis. Several studies have shown that zinc given by mouth provides some relief. Calcium is really important in your diet; review the information about calcium in chapter 5 on osteoporosis. Iron is a key element needed to prevent anemia, but a preliminary study indicates that when iron is taken in excess amounts it may be associated with heart attacks.

The reason for this is unclear, but this information points out that there are many things that we do not know about how minerals control the functions of the body. For this reason you must take care to avoid megadoses of any mineral until we know more about toxicity and injury to the body in excess.

Can you take too much of a given vitamin? Yes. The so-called fat-soluble vitamins A, D, E, and K cause serious disease in excess. Should you take a daily multivitamin with added trace minerals, iron, and calcium? Probably yes, and definitely yes if you are of a more advanced age. More and more information points to a need for trace minerals to maintain normal health and good vision. If you decide to take a standard multivitamin preparation daily, you should make sure that it is made by a reputable manufacturer known to your druggist and that each pill does not unreasonably exceed the daily recommended allowance. Do not load up on anyone's megavitamin regime until everyone knows it is safe and effective, including the FDA.

Nutrition is equal in importance to exercise and sleep for your health. We know that following a few basic rules will not only promote good health but will also help you live longer and feel better. While the numerous facts about proper nutrition at first seem confusing, you can simplify your life by following four basic rules:

1. Pay attention to how much you eat and exercise. Use a scale to tell you how well you are doing, and watch your weight daily.
2. Do not add salt to your food, and decrease the amount of fat you eat.
3. Eat a balanced and nutritious diet following the pyramid chart.
4. Regarding self-discipline and willpower, the buck stops with you!

15

Sleep Problems, Sex, and Intimacy

There are few things in life better than a good night's sleep. You wake up ready for the day, not dreading it, and eager to accomplish your goals. But you and I know what it's like to get up in the morning and feel like the night in bed was a waste of time. You recall that you spent the night turning and churning, trying to find a position in which your left shoulder didn't hurt, and you remember how your lower back started to twinge. You turned yet one more time and felt your nightgown twist around you, and so you arched your back to straighten it out. Then you sensed that the pillow was lumpy at the wrong spot, and you squirmed around, trying to make the right impression for your head. This went on all night and now, in the morning, you're suffering from a night of nonrejuvenating sleep.

This is arthritis at its worst: when it causes you to lose sleep, experience morning stiffness, and the gelling of muscles when you try to sit up. This is not the way to begin the day. In this chapter, we'll look at how you improve your sleep as well as the related bedroom topics of sex and intimacy.

Sleep

For 20 years I have written articles and spoken about the usefulness of waterbeds. Why? For one thing, the motion of the water keeps your muscles and joints from stiffening during the night. The heat from the waterbed also helps to reduce the pain. Even more important, waterbeds really help you to sleep better and have less stiffness each morning. Twenty years ago when I mentioned waterbeds, mothers of teenagers with arthritis raised an eyebrow, maybe smiled a little, and said, "Sure, get serious." Their teenagers with arthritis, of course, had a bright smile from ear to ear because this was the first benefit they had heard about having arthritis. Visions of 1960s hippies cavorting with total abandon for hours was in the public's mind. Most people, including my wife, felt like taking a canoe with a paddle to bed. Others suffering from motion sickness only lasted a few minutes. The plastic covers were thin, and vigorous bouncing caused more than one rupture. Watching 30 gallons of water cascade down the stairs is awesome. In fact, apartment owners refused to allow them for a while.

Most of this has changed today. I once spent an afternoon at a waterbed store, where I was astounded at how much the technology has improved in fabricating waterbeds. The beds are not only half as cheap as most mattresses and box springs, but they also offer features that far exceed anything I know. Today, waterbeds come in all sizes and shapes and have many options so you can tailor them to your likes and needs. My favorite is the Tube bed. This is a king-size bed made of thick, vinyl cylinders each about 4 inches wide, full of synthetic fibers that run longitudinally from head to foot. You fill each with water as full or tightly as desired. You can change the firmness easily, too. This means that your significant other can have his or her side of the bed as soft or as firm as desired. Even better, there are individual heat controls for each side of the bed.

I was astounded but not surprised to learn that waterbeds are now used in some mental health institutions because retarded children sleep better on them. Rehabilitation institutions as well as intensive care units of hospitals also use waterbeds to prevent bed sores. Even nurseries in some hospitals are using them.

So if you're looking for a good night's sleep, I seriously recommend you go to a waterbed store and try out a waterbed or perhaps an air mattress. A Gallup poll conducted in 1989 about waterbeds interviewed 300 users and 700 nonusers. They found that back pain and stiffness were significantly less in waterbed users than in conventional bed users. The number of waterbed users in the general population was 17 percent at that time, but almost 20 percent of people over 65 years of age use waterbeds! So waterbeds are used just as much, if not more, by senior citizens to help relieve back pain and stiffness.

Sex and Intimacy

Beds naturally remind us of another topic: sexual intimacy. Each of us has a different need for intimacy. Our attitudes develop in the course of our lifetimes, beginning in infancy. Some people grow up in families that rarely demonstrate affection, and their need for affection and sexual intimacy may be less than those from what I call "warm fuzzy families." But we are all born with the need for human warmth and touch. Doctors put the newborn infant on the mother's abdomen to be fondled and to hear the heartbeat they have heard for the previous nine months. As sterile as medicine can be, even medical experts acknowledge our need for bonding.

We each have different sexual needs, and even those individual needs may vary throughout our lives, depending on many factors: the demands made upon our time because of children, our need to work, or perhaps health problems. When the equation is complicated by chronic pain in one of the partners, communication becomes an imperative. In a partnership with your significant other the most important thing is to see that the needs of both partners are met, whatever they may be. Arthritis should not be an impediment to enjoying a loving, warm, complete relationship with your partner.

One of the major pitfalls to avoid is that the partner with arthritis feels unattractive and less desirable. The other person feels badly for the person with arthritis and is afraid that perhaps sex will create more pain. What a catch-22! Try to see the other person's point of view and make an effort to communicate your needs honestly. Your challenge will be not to lose sight of your biological needs. With less impairment, your choices for sexual satisfaction will be less limited. With major impairment, you will just have to be more creative in finding ways to satisfy your needs and those of your partner.

Sexual desire also does not disappear with age. I happen to know a rather rambunctious 75-year-old woman who complains from time to time about the lack of sex in her life, and her husband is 10 years younger than she. I think she's quite normal. But I also think it is normal for a person not to be interested in sexual activity. It is a most personal preference.

There are symptoms of arthritis that can certainly adversely affect sexual performance: stiffness, joint pain, fatigue, lack of mobility, feeling bad about yourself. There are ways to alleviate these problems. Of course, this means that a certain amount of planning must go into your encounters. Taking a hot bath is known to loosen the stiffness, so why not take a hot shower together? Taking an anti-inflammatory medicine an hour before can also help the pain. Resting in the afternoon would help the fatigue. And of course the early morning is usually not the best time for a person with arthritis to engage in any physical activity, so plan for the evening, or whatever part of the day when you are less stiff.

As far as feeling bad about yourself, think about how our society seems to be burdened with the Madison Avenue syndrome. There are many ills cursing this country because of the "sex sells" idea, including bulimia, anorexia, the proliferation of diet centers, diet pills, unnecessary plastic surgery, and so on. Please don't buy into that nonsense! When I saw my daughters looking at photos of a certain rock star, I told them that my heroine was Mother Teresa. When they admired some rail-thin model, I told them I admired Barbara Bush.

Our bodies all undergo change as we age. That is a fact that we must accept. Proper nutrition and exercise will improve our general condition, but our bodies do change. It is important that we all accept these changes. The real you inside is the person who matters. Do you have a cheerful attitude to encourage people to be around you? Do you contribute to a better world in your life? Are you a happy person inside? Do you care about the people around you despite your own pain and problems? Are you interested in satisfying your partner's needs also? Those are the qualities that make people want to be with you. Having arthritis has little to do with being able to love another human being. And don't we all want to be loved in our lives?

As far as the mechanical aspects of having intercourse, communication becomes important. The good news is that arthritis does not generally affect the areas of the body (including the brain) that allow you to enjoy sensual and sexual stimulation. In fact, a survey of patients with arthritis states that patients who had orgasms after sexual activity felt pain relief for up to six hours. It is impossible to say why this happens; perhaps chemicals are released into the system to eliminate pain, but I prefer to describe it as the "power of love." However, you need to let your partner know in advance that if you make a verbal expression of pain it does not necessarily mean that you are not interested in continuing to make love. It may be an involuntary expression and should not be misinterpreted. Once you become involved in the act, you will probably forget the pain of arthritis.

Any positions in which both partners are comfortable is medically fine. The traditional missionary position is probably not the best option for a person with arthritis by virtue of the weight of the man; or if the man has arthritis, he may have too much pressure on his knees and arms. Lying side by side seems to be a solution for many people. Some find that having the man lying behind the woman is a good approach. Others have found that having the woman in a standing position, leaning over a counter, and having her partner behind her is pleasant and less stressful, especially when hip joints are involved. The Arthritis Foundation publishes a pamphlet entitled *Living and Loving: Information about Sex,* which is a good starting point for discussion about some of the challenges of achieving a mutually satisfying sexual relationship.

Some Possible Complications

Frequently, if you have RA or lupus, you may experience Raynaud's phenomenon in which there is a diminished flow of blood to the extremities. During sexual activity, blood flow may be directed to the genital area, and you may experience increased pain in the toes or fingers. Again, a warm bath will help increase circulation. You need to be in a warm room, and if necessary wear a pair of warm socks. Go ahead, make a joke!

In Sjögren's syndrome there is diminished secretion of fluid from body surfaces. This can obviously create problems with vaginal lubrication. You can use a water-soluble lubricant, such as K–Y jelly, or products specifically marketed for vaginal lubrication. These are watery solutions, easily absorbed and unnecessary to remove.

Young men are more frequently diagnosed with ankylosing spondylitis. The general recommendations we've made apply to them too: warm baths, anti-inflammatory drugs, and so forth. It is recommended that they be underneath their partner, perhaps with a pillow for support, or use a side-by-side approach. Just be careful to find positions that do not aggravate the back problems.

Joint replacement surgery, especially for hips and knees, present very specific problems when it comes to sexual activity. You need to address this with your physician before you leave the hospital. Ask if you should abstain from sexual activity or just avoid certain positions for a certain period of time.

Sexual satisfaction can be achieved in many ways. Arthritis can make intercourse difficult. Stimulating your partner manually, orally, or with a vibrator in a caring, romantic way, can be satisfying. On the other hand, despite your feelings of affection there may be times when either you or your partner simply doesn't feel very passionate. Then you or your partner can certainly stimulate the other person and satisfy their sexual needs. Masturbation is also a healthy way of achieving the same goal. It can also reassure you of your own normal sexuality.

Having someone you love, someone with whom to share your life, has to be one of the all-time blessings of a happy life. If one of you develops a chronic disease, you will need all the affection and understanding you can muster to maintain a normal life. If you are the person with arthritis, you will need to let your mate know your feelings about sexual activity, and vice versa. If your mate has arthritis, you must reassure your mate that he or she is a desirable partner and that you love him or her and want to continue sharing that part of your life. Consideration, accommodation, sensitivity, and plain old-fashioned affection should rule if you are to truly enjoy the pleasure of each other's company.

Finally, remember also that intercourse is the first expression of love we think of; it is by no means the only possibility. When we truly love another person, there are many manifestations of affection. We hold hands, we hug, we pay attention to the other person's comments, we are gentle, we try not to hurt the other person, and in many other ways demonstrate our love and affection.

16

Assistive Devices to Help the Joys of Daily Life

Arthritis is disabling to many people, but fortunately, we have obtained recognition of our needs in the Americans with Disabilities Act (ADA) passed by Congress in 1990. ADA includes many components, but a major effect is to make public places more user friendly for you. This means that curbs will be leveled to get rid of steps, and ramps or elevators will be available near stairs.

Many devices also exist to help us, but before we review them, let me mention that the most helpful device is your own creativity. The American College of Rheumatology (ACR), in cooperation with the Lederle Laboratories, publishes an annual self-help guide, *Sharing Innovations* (P.O. Box 585, Summit, NJ 07902-0585), a compilation of creative ideas from people with arthritis. Robin May, a judge who has suffered from RA for more than 20 years, notes that not a day goes by that she doesn't look for ways to make an activity easier. For example, she wears a carpenter's apron around the house, filling the pockets with items that she'll need during the day, thereby avoiding unnecessary trips up the stairs. In addition, the pockets free her hands to hold onto the railing of the stairs. Another idea is to use a textured rubber soap mitt in the shower to prevent dropping the soap.

Here's an example of individual creativity once seen at a Japanese restaurant: The waiter saw a woman with arthritis of the hands having difficulty with her fork. He folded a piece of cardboard, placed it between the ends of two chopsticks, and secured the ends and cardboard with a rubber band. The result was a pair of chopsticks with a spring, easily squeezed together to hold food. So use your own creativity to protect joints, conserve energy, reduce fatigue, and make life a little easier.

A Review of Devices

In writing this book, I reviewed the most frequently ordered items from several large catalog companies and interviewed a few medical equipment store managers and arthritis doctors. The catalog companies included the *Sammon's Catalog* (1-800-323-5547), Sears' *Health Care* (1-800-326-1750, which marks the items that can be reimbursed by Medicare), and J. C. Penney's *Easy Living Fashions* (1-800-222-6161). I also recommend a book of self-help aids and products, *Guide to Independent Living for People with Arthritis,* published by the Arthritis Foundation and the Arthritis Health Professions Association, 1314 Spring St., N.W., Atlanta, GA 30309.

To introduce you to the major helpful devices, the following sections are arranged by activity. For each section, there is at least one name and phone number. This does not mean that they are the only places to obtain help, as there are literally hundreds of catalogs, but you do need a name and phone number to call as a starting point for assistive equipment.

Hand Tasks: Writing, Phoning, and Hygiene

Perhaps the single most important concern to most of us is working with our hands. You need to remember, though, that if you are looking for assistive devices to help you with hand motions, pick products that use as few hand and finger joints as possible to reduce pain. The ACR pamphlet *Sharing Innovations* notes: "Remember, make the product or task fit you—don't fit yourself to it!"

For writing, there are many devices in the three catalogs mentioned above for holding pencils and pens more effectively. For example, enlarged holders that fit over the pen make grasping easier and less painful. For a steadier hand, *Sammon's* has a Steady Write pencil and pen. Battery-operated pencil sharpeners are also useful.

If you use a computer, wrist and hand rest attachments for your keyboard are a must also (see chapter 12). *Sammon's* has an extensive selection of computer aids for disabled people.

If you read a lot, book holders are necessary to reduce fatigue in the hands. The Arthritis Foundations's *Guide to Independent Living for People with Arthritis* and *Sammon's Catalog* offer an amazing assortment of holders for reading in bed, in a chair, or at a desk.

Telephoning can be a real chore, not only in dialing but in holding the phone to your face. The AT&T Accessible Communication Product Center (1-800-233-1222, 2001 Rte. 46, Ste. 310, Parsippany, NJ 07054-1315) has a catalog to answer your special problems. The devices mainly help hearing- or speech-impaired people, but they also assist motion-impaired people. In addition, the company has 600 local AT&T Phone Centers to help you with any individual problems. (Call 1-800-222-3111 for the location of one near you.) There are amplifiers and, of course, speaker phones to eliminate fatigue of your arms while cradling a phone to your ear. You can also try a large-number keypad that requires minimal pressure to dial.

There are now electronic devices to open letters, lick stamps, and place the stamps on letters. Many catalogs and several upscale gadget stores such as the Sharper Image have them. Scissors are always a problem if it hurts your hand to squeeze. Spring-assisted scissors have oversize handles, allowing the user to use the whole hand. One brand, Fiskars, has a layer of shock-absorbing plastic cushion covering the handles. Rolling Scissors from Reliable Home Office (1-800-424-6255) is a rolling cutter that cuts straight lines in almost any kind of paper just by pushing the large handle to cut—there is no squeezing. The *Guide to Independent Living* also offers electric scissors, cordless and regular, among their many options.

Eating, Drinking, and Cooking

Most catalogs and books have sections on aids for eating, drinking, and cooking. They offer several kinds of cutlery products that are lightweight and maneuverable, featuring proper handle angles for distribution of pressure. Combination cutlery is a combination fork/knife and spoon/knife. Weighted style cutlery provides proper balance for users with limited strength. Another style of cutlery is designed to be used with the thumb opposite the index finger. Lightweight angled style cutlery has 45- and 90-degree angles for forks and spoons to make eating easier for both right- and left-handed users with limited elbow or wrist motion. Household knives have handles like pistol grips to economize effort by transferring the cutting power from the arm to the center of the knife.

If you prefer, you can also find in books and catalogs puttylike materials that can be molded to your hand to make gripping utensils better. These are recommended by many workers in the field.

Consider also an electric can opener. To open bottles, you will have to try the many types to see which one works best for you. An interesting one to me is the OpenUp electric jar opener in the Hammacher Schlemmer catalog (1-800-543-3366) that twists lids off in seconds and attaches to the wall; it has a cone-shaped grip with up to five times the twisting power of a normal hand. In short, you will find many kitchen aids in these catalogs, and so you will need to review them to see which ones help you.

Getting Dressed

The *Guide to Independent Living* lists at least 46 catalogs that offer adaptive clothing for people with disabilities. Most are devoted to women's clothing. J. C. Penney's *Easy Living Fashions* offers fashionable clothes that use Velcro instead of buttons or zippers for closure, soft elasticized waists, and sturdy fabric pull loops to give more leverage. Jackets and tops have roomier armholes for easier sliding on and off.

You can also find undergarments that have front openings and closings using Velcro or hooks as closures. One-size stretch bras offer another option to fasteners and hooks. Some undergarments offer zippers that can be zipped with one hand.

Many catalogs offer dressing aids that include large and small buttoners and unbuttoners, zipper openers, dressing sticks with garterlike clasps to hold clothing in place while dressing, apron hoops, and sock or shoe aids. The apron hoop is a bendable piece of plastic that springs back in place and is ideal around the waist to hold pants or skirts in place. A major improvement in the past several years has been the elastic shoelace that allows you to slip your shoes off and on without having to tie or untie them. Many other shoe manufacturers now make Velcro straps to fasten shoes as another option.

Bathing and Hygiene

If you are limited in function, pay a visit to a medical equipment store to see items in the bathroom category such as tubs and toilets. Alternatively, the Sears *Health Care* catalog and the *Guide to Independent Living* offer some selections, but when I visited a Sears store, I found that they refer you to the catalog and do not have a special section for health care.

Grooming and bathing aids such as comb holders, special curved brushes, safety rails, seats for the tub, Interplak electric toothbrushes, special squeeze containers for toothpaste, and special nail clippers are most completely described in the *Guide to Independent Living.*

Home Accessories and Housekeeping

One of my pharmacist friends tells me that he uses a product called Easy Dose pill splitter from Apothecary Products, Inc., 11531 Rupp Drive, Burnsville, MN 55337, (612-890-1940), for splitting pills for customers who are unable to cut the pills. This item is not expensive and is easy to use, so you might get one for yourself. The same company sells an Easy Dose pill crusher that has a spoon in the well and a round metal crusher that is pushed onto the pill.

Sammon's has a pill-cap opener to make it easy to open those ridiculous child-proof plastic bottle caps if a grandchild is not around to do so. The same catalog has a large selection of doorknob turners, scissors, special brushes for all kinds of housework, and key holders and turners. A plastic product called Dyna-Form-It, used right out of the can, easily molds into customized grips on almost anything and is particularly useful for combs, keys, eating utensils, and doorknobs.

Many people also like reachers, one of the most frequently used home accessories. These are long rods with open-jaw pincers on one end to grasp an object and are usually made of aluminum or stiff plastic with pistol-like handles and trigger designed to allow you to squeeze the trigger and securely grasp and hold onto objects. People with arthritis find them useful because it is painful to bend over to pick something up or too dangerous to get on a stool or ladder to reach up high. Many catalogs have extensive models from which to choose.

Mobility Aids

Canes, crutches, walkers, wheelchairs, and tri-wheeler power chairs are the principle mobility aids for people seriously affected by arthritis. Canes are probably the most commonly used aid-to-daily-living devices. If you have a problem with one leg, the use of a cane to take some of the weight off that leg improves mobility and reduces pain. It is important to remember that the cane is held in the hand *opposite to the painful leg.* When walking, the cane is extended when the bad leg is bearing the weight of walking. This may seem too obvious, but people often use a cane on the same side time after time. The height of the cane is also important; it should be long enough that your elbow is almost straight when you are leaning on it. A single rubber-tipped cane is the most commonly used. Equipment store managers told me, however, that most people buy a quad cane. This is a cane with a pod of four tips, which provides greater stability when walking. The cane comes in two styles, wide and narrow. The narrow size has the tips closer together in the pod so that walking up stairs is easier. There is also a tripod cane, which is not sold as often.

You may need crutches when both legs have problems or one leg has such pain that weight bearing is undesirable or impossible. Sometimes you can use only one crutch, but usually two crutches are better. If your hands are painful, use the platform crutch, which has an arm-rest forearm support that allows easier motion. Crutches should be carefully measured by a qualified person. Your elbows should be barely bent when you place your hands in the hand grips and are bearing weight. The underarm pads must be lower than the underarm, and you must not lean on the crutch when walking. Your hands must bear the weight. Be sure to have a rubber tip on your crutch point to prevent you from slipping. In the catalogs already mentioned a wide variety of crutch accessories are available.

Walkers can help many people who are too weak to support weight or who need more stability. These devices have four legs, are built of lightweight metal, and form a supporting frame around the user. The height of a walker must be set so that the elbow is bent and able to pick up the walker to make the next step. Most walkers have wheels in front and rubber tipped legs in back for easier walking and maneuverability; four-wheel walkers are rarely used. Most catalogs offer a variety of walker accessories, such as pouches to store needed items.

Wheelchairs need to be individually fitted if you are going to require one for a long time. The expertise needed cannot be provided by a catalog. You will need to be properly measured and fitted at an equipment store. If you can afford it, an electric wheelchair or tri-wheeler adds enormously to mobility.

Driving and Transportation

In years past, people with serious arthritis were unable to get out and be independent. Now quite a few devices are available to allow you to continue independent living. Often the biggest problem is opening the car door and turning on the ignition. Special devices are available to allow you to do this. The Arthritis Foundation's *Guide to Independent Living* contains the best discussion of driving and transportation needs and equipment.

Don't let your arthritis prevent you from enjoying life. Whatever your problem, you can most likely find a device that will enable you to continue living a full and joyous life.

Part Four

PAYING ATTENTION

TO YOUR

SPECIAL ISSUES

17

On the Job with Arthritis

Employment for most of us is essential if we want to pay our bills and live well. People with arthritis are no exception. Having arthritis definitely adds to your challenge not only to find a job but to keep it. In this chapter, we'll focus on a few major issues that may help you, including how to apply for a job, how to adapt to your job, and changing jobs.

Applying for a Job

You have arthritis and are able to work; you have a skill and with a little help from assistive devices you can do it with the best of them. How do you handle the application and interview? Should you tell the employer that you have arthritis? Should you apply to a big company, or should you stick to a with a mid- or small-sized company?

For answers to these and other questions, I interviewed several personnel directors of large and small companies. In addition, I talked to insurance agents and people on the job with arthritis. The replies were surprising but not unexpected.

Until the health insurance system is changed in our country, you need to apply to a large company with more than a hundred employees and preferably thousands of employees if you want career growth. Your ability to change jobs is limited because of probable health insurance penalties, so you need to be in a company large enough for you to expand your horizons. Another reason is that larger companies are often self-insured with stop-loss backup insurance to protect themselves, so they are more willing to take a risk with you and let your fellow employees subsidize your potentially more expensive health-care needs. On the other hand, you need to be careful because many self-insured plans are not subject to state insurance laws, and so these companies can make discriminatory rules to exclude your disease from coverage. But in general, the bigger the company, the less likely it is to exclude your arthritis.

In companies with fewer than a hundred employees, an insurance-block pool of many small companies is a common way of providing health insurance coverage. Employees are placed in groups of 10 by the insurers and based on the information gathered in the application, they may decide to cover nine people and exclude one with arthritis. You might say, "Don't tell them on the application. Who's to know the difference?" However, insurance carriers have a Medical Information Bureau (MIB) that pools information from many companies about health-care risks. If they discover that you have falsified information, you can be excluded from all further coverage, despite rules prohibiting exclusion on the basis of disease in most states.

According to one personnel director of a large company, here is the best way to handle this: Unless the interviewer asks specifically about your health problems, don't bring your arthritis up. After you have the job and you are asked to fill out a health insurance form, the question about prior illness will be on the application, so tell the truth then. Do not lie at this point.

With the rising cost of health insurance, the most recent trend by employers is to reduce benefits to cut down the amount paid in premiums. The present reductions include eliminating paying for prescriptions and dropping dental insurance. Unfortunately, as long as premiums rise 10 to 20 percent per year, and our insurance system is not changed, you will see more and more reductions of services, and more rationing of care will occur for chronically ill people.

If your company offers life insurance as a benefit, grab it and keep it. As a person with arthritis, you are considered a high risk, and getting life insurance on your own will either be very expensive or nearly impossible.

Adapting to the Workplace

Most employers are sympathetic to your needs for some help in doing your work efficiently. Some rheumatologists ask you to wear wrist-resting splints if you do clerical work and have arthritis of the hands or wrists. If you use a computer or typewriter, you certainly need keyboard hand rests. Use an adjustable-height chair to give your back, arms, and legs a rest by changing the chair's height frequently. Don't forget to get up and move around every 20 to 30 minutes to keep inactivity stiffness at bay. You will more than likely have no difficulty in being allowed to move around to lessen stiffness—everyone needs to do this. The Arthritis Foundation's *Guide to Independent Living* has an excellent section on vocational aids in the workplace if you need more adaptation.

Another vexing problem for employees is tardiness due to stiffness or pain in the morning, or needing to rest after lunch. If you have this problem, arrange to stay later or make up the time. If you need time off to get tests done or see your doctor, offer to make up the time. Do not abuse the system, as it makes it more difficult for others with arthritis to be treated fairly and sensitively.

Changing Jobs

You've done the best you can, but the demands of your job are simply more than you can handle in spite of assistive devices and an understanding boss. Before you decide to change jobs, though, see if your company has another job that they would consider retraining you to do. Large companies would rather keep an old employee if possible because it's cheaper to retrain someone who knows the organization than to bring in a new person. If this option is not open for you, visit the vocational rehabilitation service in your city. In Texas, they're pretty good about helping someone who wants help. Some chapters of the Arthritis Foundation have vocational counseling groups to advise you.

Finally, let me pass on a lesson I've learned over the past few years. Most of us worry about pleasing others and whether our efforts are OK. There is an old saying that the moment of inner contentment and greater success comes when we accept that we are acceptable. For people with arthritis trying to keep a job or get a job, attitude and poise in adversity are essential. Knowing that you are acceptable not only to yourself but to others and to society goes a long way in helping not only you but the people around you.

18

Deciding Whether You Should Try Surgery

One of the truly great advances in the treatment of arthritis has been in orthopedic surgery. In the past, when hips or knees were so painful or so limited in motion that getting around was impossible, the arthritis sufferer was doomed to a lifetime in bed. Now, with the development of joint replacement, a new life has opened to these previously infirm people. The results are not hype, they're real. In addition to joint replacement, there are several other helpful procedures such as *synovectomy* (removal of diseased tissue from the joint), reconstruction of a joint, or fusion of a joint. We'll discuss all of your options in this chapter.

Basic Issues

Surgery in people with arthritis should not be viewed as a last resort becasue it actually serves two purposes. The first major purpose of surgery is to correct something that is wrong. For example, serious injury to a joint or tendon by such common diseases as RA or OA forces consideration of surgical efforts to relieve unremitting pain, improve motion or function, or correct deformities. But a second major purpose of surgery is to prevent further injury by an operation. Synovectomy (removal of diseased tissue inside of a joint) is an example.

In deciding whether to go through with an operation for a particular problem, you need to consider the basic disease as well as the injury itself. In the knee, for example, when the progression of serious joint injury has occurred to the point that bone is grinding on bone with each step, you would think that it doesn't make any real difference whether the initial problem was due to trauma, RA, or OA. It does. If the cause is trauma or OA, the disease has already done whatever damage it's going to do, and replacement of the joint or other procedure is worthwhile. But with RA, the inflammation can return any time and cause further damage even after an operation is done, and so the disease itself is an added consideration.

The expectations of an individual with serious arthritis can be unrealistic or excessive. It is essential that you know in great detail what you can expect and what is the down side. Your attitude about not only the surgery but life itself has an important bearing on a decision whether or not to undergo surgery. If you are depressed and weak, efforts to overcome both are needed before you undergo the surgery.

Start by thinking about what you want to get if the surgery is successful. The best outcome, of course, is relief of pain, but so is improvement in the quality of your life and life-style. Will you get an improvement in function that will allow you more freedom to do things and require less help from others? In this day of very expensive health insurance for people with arthritis or other chronic illness, you must realistically assess the benefit against the cost. This includes finding out whether or how much your insurance will cover *before* and not *after* the procedure. You will also need to establish a home support system for weeks or even months, and that too can be costly.

Selecting Your Orthopedist

Orthopedists not only pioneered the highly effective joint replacement techniques but they have been for years at the forefront of developing coordinated team care for people with chronic illness. They were working hand in hand, providing team care with physical therapists, brace people, occupational therapists, and nurses long before other fields of medicine recognized the value of this, including arthritis doctors. Orthopedists have also been pioneers in patient education, teaching patients about their illnesses and operations.

In all likelihood, your personal doctor will recommend an orthopedist to you. The probability is that the two of them work together well, and your doctor feels that the orthopedist will do the best job for you. Because your problem is highly specialized, the orthopedist is best equipped to handle it. However, be sure that she or he is board certified or at least board eligible. Find out what hospital he or she uses for surgery to be sure it meets your standards. Ask friends connected with the medical profession about the orthopedist. Calling the local medical society office is usually not helpful except to learn whether he or she is a member in good standing.

When you visit the orthopedist for the first time, judge whether he or she takes the time to explain what is wrong and what can be done to help. *Do not be shy about asking questions.* If you don't like the doctor or your personalities don't mesh, find someone else. Be sure that you get some printed material to review from the doctor, or that a nurse sits with you to explain what will happen. Ultimately though, trust your own instinct to use this doctor or not.

Major Types of Operations

Following are three major types of operations performed today:

Joint replacement. Developed in the 1960s, replacement of badly diseased arthritic hips was done with a metal hip-joint–shaped device wedged into the thigh bone with a synthetic cushion attached to the acetabulum (cup of the pelvis) to absorb pressure and shock. Joint replacement has opened a whole new world to literally hundreds of thousands of people otherwise limited to a wheelchair or bedridden existence. Improvements in the materials have also allowed replacement or partial replacement of knees, finger joints, elbows, shoulders, and other joints. The main complications of this surgery include infection and the loosening of the shaft of the prosthesis embedded in the center of the thigh bone. However, relief of pain and improvement of motion occur in 9 out of 10 people receiving the hip procedure, so your risk of failure is low.

Synovectomy. This operation removes inflamed lining tissue from the inside of the joint. The concept of this operation is that joint injury will be reduced by removing the diseased tissue. An added benefit is that your severe pain will usually go away. The knee is probably the most frequent site for this type of operation. Entry into the joint is either by an open incision or through the arthroscope, a widely used flexible tube instrument that allows the orthopedist not only to see inside the joint but to remove tissue through a tiny incision in the skin.

Fusion and Resection. Fusion is an example of a preventive operation. An example is fusion of neck vertebrae to make the neck stronger when arthritis has destroyed too much bone in critical places. If not done, pain is severe, and there is risk of injury to the nerves in the neck. The removal or resection of bones to provide relief from pain is useful. An example is the removal of the heads of the bones in the ball of the foot when they are seriously injured by arthritis and are painful to stand or walk on.

Getting Ready for Surgery

If you and your doctor have concluded that all medical treatments have been unsuccessful in controlling pain, or that your motion and function are so restricted that your quality of life is altered, surgery such as a joint replacement is necessary.

This is a team effort and starts with your arthritis doctor and orthopedist working with you as members of a team to be sure that you are in the best condition possible to go to surgery. Be sure that the rest of the team—nurse, physical therapist, educator, and others—are on board and coordinating the necessary activities.

One of the first things you need to do is to review your medicines with your own doctor and with the orthopedist as well. Many orthopedists want your prednisone level as low as possible, then add a boost at the time of surgery to help the adrenal gland with stress reaction. Infection may be more frequent in patients on steroids. If you are on NSAIDs, the doctor will usually halt their use for a while before surgery because bleeding can be a problem in people taking NSAIDs. Some orthopedists also believe that d-penicillamine can delay healing. So you can see how important it is to review all of your medicines. (If you are taking any medicines prescribed by another doctor, it's important for your orthopedist to know.) The doctor will try to get rid of any known minor infections before surgery. Examples are carious teeth (tooth decay) or inflamed gums, low-grade urinary tract infections, or infection of the prostate gland.

If at all possible, you should also have a planned program of exercise to strengthen the muscles around the hip or whatever joint is being operated on. Success is much greater with better endurance and strength. General fitness, as we have discussed earlier in several sections of the book, is even more important here.

Above all, nothing is more important than keeping a positive attitude toward what will be a painful procedure. You have to remember that the relief of pain and increased function will be worth it. You must be prepared mentally to do whatever is needed following your operation even though you will hurt. For example, if you don't exercise, the muscles will stiffen, and your results will be less effective. If you are unwilling to do this, you probably should not have the operation. It is that important.

After Surgery

You will need several weeks to recuperate. There will be pain, and when your doctor tells you that it's time to move the painful joints, you won't believe it. After my wife had surgery to her shoulder, she extended her arm, and walked her fingers up the wall to get motion back in her shoulder with tears in her eyes. But she has nearly full motion in her shoulder now. Before you undergo surgery, make up your mind that even though there is pain, you will do the exercises that the orthopedist and physical therapist ask you to do.

Be sure that you have your home support team in place before going home. You'll need someone to drive you to appointments, for example. Have a written plan from the team at the hospital and the name of a designated person to be your liaison to the doctor and community-based services such as physical therapy. Remember what we've discussed about exercise (chapter 13) and check with your doctor and team as to when you can start with your exercise program again.

Orthopedic surgery offers great benefits to people with arthritis. Surgery is done for two reasons: (1) to correct a diseased joint to reduce pain, improve motion, or correct deformities (joint replacement is the most successful example); and (2) to prevent or reduce further disease, such as a back operation to remove bone that is impinging on nerves.

Before an operation, you need to be sure that your expectations are in line with what is realistic. Your attitude must be positive, and you must be ready to accept pain after the surgery. Exercise is even more important after surgery than before surgery. You must be sure that your health insurance will cover you. You can no longer assume that an insurance carrier will cover "anything."

Joint replacement has brought enormous joy to the lives of thousands of arthritis sufferers by eliminating pain and improving motion. This allows the person with arthritis to be mobile and enjoy independent living.

19

Pregnancy and Arthritis

The main questions in the minds of women with arthritis regarding pregnancy are:

- Is it possible to become pregnant?
- How much trouble will I have during pregnancy?
- Will the baby be OK?
- What do I do about my medicines?
- Will my baby have arthritis?
- Will I have trouble taking care of the baby?
- Can I nurse my baby?

Let's address each concern individually. This is one of the few situations in which the kind of arthritis you have makes a difference in what may happen. We'll only talk about two of the main kinds of arthritis that give difficulty during pregnancy: rheumatoid arthritis and systemic lupus erythematosus. A detailed discussion of the other arthritic illnesses such as ankylosing spondylitis will not be provided here because most women experience little trouble during pregnancy with these forms.

Is It Possible to Become Pregnant?

Yes, indeed, it's not only possible but probable that you can become pregnant. There is no loss of fertility because of RA or SLE. However, not feeling well or being in poor physical shape because of illness reduces your ability to get pregnant, so you'll need to do a few things before getting pregnant, which we'll review below.

How Much Trouble Will I Have During Pregnancy?

One of the nice things about RA is that many, if not most women, have a complete or almost complete remission during the early months of pregnancy that lasts until six weeks or so after delivery. This, of course, simplifies your need for medicines that may harm the fetus. It's impressive to see swollen and painful joints melt away to be normal and pain-free. But keep in mind that sometimes the remission doesn't come. No one knows why remission occurs with pregnancy, but it does.

SLE is a different story, though, as pregnancy increases the chance that the disease may worsen, causing high blood pressure, fluid retention, and even seizures. Miscarriages and premature births occur more frequently in mothers with SLE. In addition, if kidney or heart disease complicates your case, you may have a serious problem. Having related this, however, let us add that many women with SLE have normal babies. You and your doctor must decide how safe it really is for you to become pregnant.

Will My Baby Be OK?

In general, babies of RA mothers are no more likely to have birth defects or prematurity than babies of any other mother. This is not the case in SLE. Some babies have neonatal lupus, where a rash of lupus is present with positive blood tests, although this usually goes away in a few months. However, the baby's heart can be affected for reasons that are not clear, and congenital heart block (a block of the electrical impulses running through the heart muscle that activate the heartbeat) can occur, requiring a pacemaker.

What Do I Do About My Medicines?

This is a tough problem for you and your doctor and will require planning together. Most of the medicines used to treat RA can cause difficulty for the fetus or the mother. What makes it easier is that you will probably have a remission by the fourth month of pregnancy and won't need much, if any, medications. However, the major injury to babies occurs in the first three months of pregnancy; hence, the dilemma. Let's talk about the various medicines and outline the dangers you need to consider.

Aspirin and the other NSAIDs are the most commonly used medicines for arthritis, as you know. They can cause bleeding of the placenta, prolonged labor, and anemia in the mother. NSAIDs cross the placental barrier and can cause bleeding in the fetus. Dr.

Robert Zurier of Worcester, Massachusetts, feels that NSAIDs, including aspirin, have not been studied sufficiently in pregnancy and should not be considered safe. Aspirin also is not recommended for nursing mothers, as it shows up in the breast milk. When absolutely necessary, a few of the NSAIDs such as ibuprofen (Advil, and others) have a short half-life in the blood and can be used while breast-feeding.

Hydroxychloroquine (Plaquenil) is one of the antimalarial drugs used in arthritis. Because it crosses the placenta and may affect the eye, its use in pregnancy is not recommended.

Gold salts are not known to produce congenital defects with any frequency, but in theory problems could occur. A practical problem is that it takes four to six months to rid the body of gold, so if you become pregnant while on gold, it does little good to suddenly stop. If gold does cause problems, the worst time for exposure is in the first trimester of pregnancy, so you should stop gold medications several months before becoming pregnant. In my experience, gold salts do not cause much if any trouble in pregnancy, but I still recommend avoidance.

Methotrexate is rapidly becoming one of the leading medicines for RA. However, it has the unfortunate risk of producing increased numbers of birth defects and miscarriages and is excreted in breast milk in small quantities. These problems do not occur if methotrexate is discontinued prior to conception. Sulfasalazine (Azulfidine) is also used in people with inflammatory bowel disease, but the risk of birth defects resulting from this appear to be low. Pencillamine is thought to be potentially risky to the fetus, but there are not enough data to evaluate the situation conclusively.

Two cancer drugs that are used in smaller doses for RA, azathioprine and cyclophosphamide, can both cause birth defects and suppression of the immune system. Cyclophosphamide is more effective but also poses the highest risk.

Perhaps the most useful medication is prednisone, which most rheumatologists that I know prescribe in low doses during pregnancy. The risk of birth defects and miscarriage is thought to be minimal to none from this drug.

When you have decided to conceive, to help minimize risks you should discuss with your doctor a plan to discontinue medications well before becoming pregnant, at least three months. You may experience painful flares unless you begin low-dose prednisone and stop your other medications. If you take gold, you will need to stop several months before you try to conceive; the NSAIDs can be stopped a week or so before conception. Penicillamine and hydroxychloroquine accumulate in the tissues and should also be stopped early.

In SLE sufferers the situation is different. A serious flare is likely, and you and your doctor will have to balance your own health against the risk to the fetus. Again, many mothers have successful pregnancies and normal babies, but prudence is crucial in this important decision.

Will My Baby Have Arthritis?

Probably not. While women who are RF positive have a genetic predisposition to RA, few of their children develop arthritis in the childhood years. Putting it into perspective, the chances of your baby dying of an injury, accident, or some other serious illness are much greater than their getting RA in childhood. There is a greater likelihood, though, that these children will develop RA at some point during their lives.

The same is true for lupus. Few children of mothers with SLE ever have the disease during childhood years. There is a genetic predisposition, and in some ethnic groups such as African-American and Asian-American, the chances of disease at some time in life is far greater. As already mentioned, babies at birth can have neonatal lupus, due to transfer of maternal disease antibodies, but this only lasts a few weeks or months.

Will I Have Trouble Taking Care of My Baby?

For the first month or two, performing your motherly duties will be easy because you will most likely still be in remission. After that, however, the flare of RA can be worse than before. You and your doctor will need to plan when to start taking the old medicines again. If you had little disability before pregnancy, you probably will have few problems. If you had significant problems, you need to plan and decide whether your limitations are too much to handle the added burden of careing for a baby.

The work of a mother is physically more taxing than most jobs done by men. Use the information in chapter 16 about assistive devices to find some aids for you. Also, be sure to get solid support and help from your significant other. I recommend the Arthritis Foundation book, *Guide to Independent Living*, for its excellent information on this topic.

Can I Nurse My Baby?

Of course, but be sure to stay on low-dose prednisone or consult your doctor about drugs, since many, such as NSAIDs, are excreted in small amounts in the breast milk. Many other medicines involve some risk, so avoid them if you are breast-feeding. If you must take the other medicines, you probably should consider using bottled milk for the baby. This is more of a problem for mothers with SLE.

A Note from Kathy

As the woman author of this team, let me add that the decision to have a baby is one of the most important life-altering decisions a woman will have to make. The desire to have children is a tremendous drive within us: Mother Nature's way of continuing the species. If you are a woman with one of the many forms of arthritis, pregnancy becomes a little more complicated than it would be normally. The good news is that having arthritis does not generally affect your ability to conceive and carry a child to term. As Earl said, many women report that their arthritis, especially rheumatoid arthritis, subsides considerably while they are pregnant, although researchers don't yet know why.

The bad news is that you will have to do a little more forward planning than a woman without arthritis. Some of the issues that you will need to address are the effect of medications on your unborn baby, the effect on your body of stopping or decreasing the dosage of medications, and your ability to care for the child when it is born. If you have serious impairments from your arthritis, you will have to have help with the baby. Being a mother is a very physical thing. A very dear friend of mine had to seriously examine this situation, but it was due to a very different problem. She had polio as a child and now has to walk with arm-braced crutches. When she and her husband decided to have children, they both knew that it would be impossible for her to carry a child any distance at all. Together they decided that a family would be worth the extra effort it would require on both their parts. Even though she cannot walk without crutches, and she drives her car with a hand control, she has four beautiful children. Sure, the family had to make sacrifices in budgeting for extra help when the children were small, but I assure you that they consider such sacrifices well worth it. These are very personal decisions and they need to be made mutually, in an intelligent manner, looking at the future as well as the present.

So if you've decided to have a child, here's what I recommend. First, introduce your rheumatologist to your obstetrician. They will have to work closely with you to organize the birth of a healthy baby. That is the mission. For about one year you will need to gear your life to creating the healthiest newborn you can. Every pregnant woman needs to be concerned about good nutrition, taking the proper vitamins, *not drinking alcohol,* getting adequate rest, and keeping stress to a minimum.

As a mother-to-be with arthritis, you will have a few extra concerns. As Earl said, you need to consult with your doctor about which medications will have an effect on your unborn baby, and then you'll have to stop using them. But there are other issues too. For example, the hot bath that was recommended for you as a person with arthritis is no longer recommended for you as a pregnant woman. As of August 1992, pregnant women are warned that taking a hot bath, as well as sitting in a hot tub or sauna, in the first three months of pregnancy may increase the incidence of birth defects in newborns.

The physical changes that take place during pregnancy may also have an impact on your arthritis. Of course you will gain weight, and extra weight will mean extra pressure on your joints. Although too much weight gain can be detrimental, too little weight gain could mean that you and the baby are not getting proper nourishment. So balance your needs.

The commonsense approach is to continue to exercise to keep

your muscles strong and your joints flexible. A brisk walk or a swim each day will do nicely. You need to eat a proper diet not only to keep your weight within normal limits, but also to have a wonderful, healthy baby. During pregnancy, joints tend to become looser in preparation for the delivery. In later months you might have increased water retention, which may increase stiffness. All of the above problems can be dealt with in conjunction with your physicians.

With any pregnancy the hormone level is rather like a thunderstorm and you can be extremely volatile, laughing one minute and crying the next. Your emotions play a big part in your general health and you will have to find ways to reduce some of the emotional stress by finding ways to relax.

The Arthritis Foundation has a pamphlet called *Arthritis and Pregnancy,* which gives some terrific tips on organizing your life after the baby arrives, including bathing, feeding, lifting, and carrying. I am sure you can also find some really creative ways to have a happy, normal motherhood. Good luck!

Appendix 1

National Arthritis Organizations

The Arthritis Foundation
Spring St.
Atlanta, Georgia 30309
404-872-7100

Ankylosing Spondylitis Association
511 N. La Cienega
Los Angeles, California 90048
1-800-777-8189

Lupus Foundation of America
Massachusetts Ave. N.W., Ste. 203
Washington, DC 20036
202-328-4550

Scleroderma Federation
1725 York Ave. #29F
New York, New York 10128
212-427-7040

Sjögren's Syndrome Foundation
29 Gateway Dr.
Great Neck, New York 11021
516-487-2243

Appendix 2

Local Arthritis Foundation Chapters

Alabama Chapter
Birmingham, Alabama
205-979-5700

South Alabama Chapter
Mobile, Alabama
205-432-7171

Alaska Unit
Anchorage, Alaska
916-924-1878

Central Arizona Chapter
Phoenix, Arizona
602-264-7679

Southern Arizona Chapter
Tucson, Arizona
602-290-9090

Arkansas Chapter
Little Rock, Arkansas
501-664-7242

Northeastern California Chapter
Sacramento, California
916-921-5533

Northern California Chapter
San Francisco, California
415-673-6882

San Diego Area Chapter
San Diego, California
619-492-1090

Southern California Chapter
Los Angeles, California
213-938-6111

Rocky Mountain Chapter
Denver, Colorado
303-756-8622

Connecticut Chapter
Rocky Hill, Connecticut
203-563-1177

Delaware Chapter
Wilmington, Delaware
302-764-8254

Florida Chapter
Bradenton, Florida
813-795-3010

Georgia Chapter
Atlanta, Georgia
404-351-0454

Hawaii Chapter
Honolulu, Hawaii
808-235-3636

Idaho Chapter
Boise, Idaho
208-344-7102

Illinois Chapter
Chicago, Illinois
312-782-1367

Central Illinois Chapter
Peoria, Illinois
309-682-6600

Indiana Chapter
Indianapolis, Indiana
317-879-0321

Iowa Chapter
Des Moines, Iowa
515-278-0636

Kansas Chapter
Wichita, Kansas
316-263-0116

Kentucky Chapter
Louisville, Kentucky
502-893-9771

Louisiana Chapter
Baton Rouge, Louisiana
504-387-6932

Maine Chapter
Brunswick, Maine
207-773-0595

Maryland Chapter
Lutherville, Maryland
410-561-8090

Massachusetts Chapter
Newton, Massachusetts
617-244-1800

Michigan Chapter
Southfield, Michigan
313-350-3030

Minnesota Chapter
Minneapolis, Minnesota
612-874-1201

Mississippi Chapter
Jackson, Mississippi
601-956-3371

Eastern Missouri Chapter
St. Louis, Missouri
314-644-3488

Western Missouri–Greater Kansas City Chapter
Kansas City, Missouri
816-361-7002

Montana Chapter
National Office
404-872-7100

Nebraska Chapter
Omaha, Nebraska
402-391-8000

Nevada Chapter
Las Vegas, Nevada
702-367-1626

New Hampshire Chapter
Concord, New Hampshire
603-244-9322

New Jersey Chapter
Iselin, New Jersey
908-283-4300

New Mexico Chapter
Albuquerque, New Mexico
505-265-1545

Central New York Chapter
Syracuse, New York
315-455-8553

Genesee Valley Chapter
Rochester, New York
716-423-9490

Long Island Chapter
Melville, New York
516-427-8272

New York Chapter
New York, New York
212-477-8310

Northeastern New York Chapter
Albany, New York
518-459-1203

Western New York Chapter
Tonawanda, New York
716-837-8600

North Carolina Chapter
Durham, North Carolina
919-596-3360

Dakota Chapter
Fargo, North Dakota
701-237-3310

Central Ohio Chapter
Columbus, Ohio
614-488-0777

Northeastern Ohio Chapter
Beachwood, Ohio
216-831-7000

Northwestern Ohio Chapter
Toledo, Ohio
419-537-0888

Southwestern Ohio Chapter
Cincinnati, Ohio
513-271-4545

Eastern Oklahoma Chapter
Tulsa, Oklahoma
918-743-4526

Oklahoma Chapter
Oklahoma City, Oklahoma
405-521-0066

Oregon Chapter
Portland, Oregon
503-222-7246

Central Pennsylvania Chapter
Camp Hill, Pennsylvania
717-763-0900

Eastern Pennsylvania Chapter
Philadelphia, Pennsylvania
215-574-9480

Western Pennsylvania Chapter,
Pittsburgh, Pennsylvania
412-566-1645

Rhode Island Chapter
East Providence, Rhode Island
401-434-5792

South Carolina Chapter
Columbia, South Carolina
803-254-6702

Middle-East Tennessee Chapter
Nashville, Tennessee
615-329-3431

West Tennessee Chapter
Memphis, Tennessee
901-365-7080

North Texas Chapter
Dallas, Texas
214-826-4361

Northwest Texas Chapter
Fort Worth, Texas
817-926-7733

South Central Texas Chapter
San Antonio, Texas
512-224-8222

Texas Gulf Coast Chapter
Houston, Texas
713-785-2360

Utah Chapter
Salt Lake City, Utah
801-486-4993

Vermont 8 Northern New York Chapter
Burlington, Vermont
802-864-4988

Metropolitan Washington Chapter
Arlington, Virginia
703-276-7555

Virginia Chapter
Richmond, Virginia
804-379-7464

Washington State Chapter
Seattle, Washington
206-622-1378

Wisconsin Chapter
West Allis, Wisconsin
414-321-3933

Index